LOW BACK PAIN

An Historical and Contemporary Overview of the Occupational, Medical, and Psychosocial Issues of Chronic Back Pain

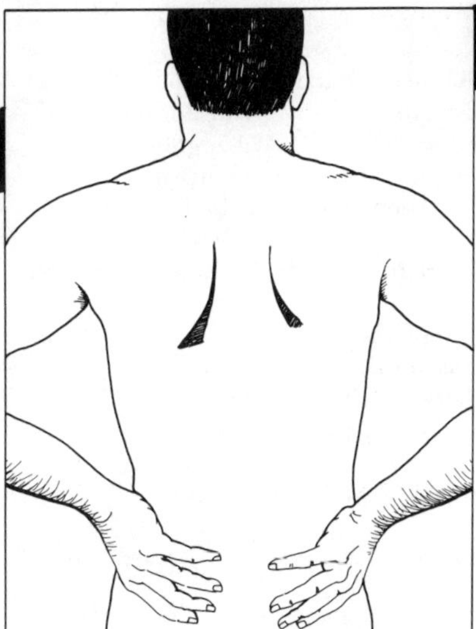

Peter Mandell MD
Marvin H Lipton MD
Joseph Bernstein MD
Gilbert J Kucera MD
Jeffrey A Kampner BA

SLACK Incorporated, 6900 Grove Road, Thorofare, New Jersey 08086

SLACK International Book Distributors

In Europe, the Middle East and Africa:
John Wiley & Sons Limited
Baffins Lane
Chichester, West Sussex P019 1UD
England

In Canada:
McAinsh and Company
2760 Old Leslie Street
Willowdale, Ontario M2K 2X5

In Australia and New Zealand:
MacLennan & Petty Pty Limited
P.O. Box 425
Artarmon, N.S.W. 2064
Australia

In Japan:
Central Foreign Books Limited
1-13 Jimbocho-Kanda
Tokyo, Japan

In Asia and India:
PG Publishing Pte Limited.
36 West Coast Road, #02-02
Singapore 0512

Foreign Translation Agent

John Scott & Company
International Publishers' Agency
417-A Pickering Road
Phoenixville, PA 19460

Publisher: Harry C. Benson
Managing Editor: Lynn Borders
Editor: Cheryl D. Willoughby
Designer: Susan Hermansen
Production Manager: David Murphy

Printed in the United States of America

Library of Congress Catalog Card Number: 89-042576

ISBN: 1-556420-82-X

Published by: SLACK Incorporated
6900 Grove Rd.
Thorofare, NJ 08086

Last digit is print number: 10 9 8 7 6 5 4 3 2 1

Authors

Peter Mandell, M.D.
Assistant Clinical Professor of
Orthopaedic Surgery, University
of California, San Francisco
Instructor in Anatomy, San Francisco
Combined Orthopaedic Residency Training Program
Associate Chief of Orthopaedic Surgery,
Mt. Zion Hospital and Medical Center,
San Francisco

Marvin H. Lipton, M.D.
Assistant Clinical Professor of
Orthopaedic Surgery, University
of California, San Francisco
Associate Chief of Orthopaedic Surgery
Mt. Zion Hospital and Medical Center,
San Francisco

Joseph Bernstein, M.D.
Assistant Clinical Professor of
Orthopaedic Surgery, University
of California, San Francisco
Associate Chief of Orthopaedic Surgery
Mt. Zion Hospital and Medical Center,
San Francisco

Gilbert J. Kucera, M.D.
Assistant Clinical Professor of
Orthopaedic Surgery, University
of California, San Francisco
Orthopaedic Consultant to the
United States Olympic Ski Team
Associate Chief of Orthopaedic Surgery
Mt. Zion Hospital and Medical Center,
San Francisco

Jeffrey A. Kampner, B.A.
Editorial Manager

Table of Contents

CHAPTER 1

Epidemiology of Low-back Pain

Introduction

The incidence and distribution of low back pain is extremely diverse. It has a pervasive influence in nearly every existing occupation, affecting 75 to 80 million Americans at a cost of $30 billion per year in lost production, sickness benefits and treatment. In terms of human cost, fully 1% of the population is considered "totally and permanently" disabled by chronic back problems, with many more partially disabled [1]. Low back pain is reported to be the most common type of chronic pain and the number one compensable disability [2]. According to the National Center for Health Statistics, back and spine impairments are the most common causes of activity limitation in persons less than 45 years old [3]. Discogenic problems ranked as the 11th most frequent reason for days of hospitalization in the U.S. and as the number one reason in 13 states [4]. Back pain is the number one reason for physician contact in this country [5]. In Sweden, low back pain is the leading cause of worker absenteeism and compensation claims, as manifested from 1955 to 1971, when 31% of all Swedish citizens and 46% of non-Swedish citizens had at some point missed work [6].

With the widely-accepted finding that nearly 80% of all human beings will be affected by low back pain at some point in life (those between 50 and 60 having a 70% chance of chronic pain), the syndrome of backache does not discriminate against sex, race or work environment, although some groups are more susceptible to pathology than others [7]. There is a remarkable similarity in the number of low-back injuries as a percentage of all reportable occupational injuries between Great Britain (27%), Ontario (23%), and the United States (26-29%) [8]. These rates have shown very little variation through the years. Others report finding 10-15% of these populations experiencing back pain every year [9].

Yet these alarming numbers are deceptive because low-back pain is usually a self-limiting condition, where recovery without a physician's consultation can be demonstrated in 80-90% of all episodes. In fact, the literature is in basic agreement that 80-90% of all cases improve within eight weeks, regardless of treatment [7,9,10]. According to Steinberg, 97% of patients avoid hospitalization and 99.5% circumvent surgery, while Horal has indicated that only 2.4% of controls and 4% of sick-listed patients had a low-back pain condition in excess of six months duration [7,10]. Despite the capability of the lumbar spine to heal itself, the reason the problem of backache remains universally pervasive is the widely accepted fact that the recurrence rate is just as high (if not higher) than the initial incidence rate. Furthermore, the relatively few chronic cases that do not heal within two months account for nearly three times more work days lost, restricted activity, and disability [11].

The high incidence and prevalence of low back pain has led to research in three primary epidemiologic categories: environmental, physiological and psychosocial risk factors. Most epidemiological studies have evaluated environmental stresses experienced in the work place. Those jobs that entail a significant degree of lifting, bending, twisting, work standardization and monotony, sitting and standing correlate with a greater incidence of low back pain in many recent studies. Physiological risk factors include sex, height, weight, other anthropometric characteristics and physical fitness. Finally, particular psychosocial factors are associated with higher levels of chronic back pain, including emotional distress, increased bodily awareness, neuroticism, job satisfaction, job security, education, social isolation and decreased ego strength, a pain-oriented personality, hostility towards medical care, alcoholism and drug dependency.

Steinberg compared a review of epidemiological research to "eating popovers – one has to bite into and chew up a lot of hot air in order to get something solid to swallow" [7]. This chapter will try to distinguish "edible" information from the synthetic substitutes which often only validate an investigators preconceived prejudices. Our objective is twofold: to explain which occupations are most hazardous to the health of the spine, and what causative factors are responsible. What follows is a diverse assortment of statistics, results, observations and opinions taken from current medical literature, ranging from studies on interstate bus drivers to helicopter pilots to concrete reinforcement workers. We feel these articles are indicative of mainstream epidemiological research.

Many observations will come into conflict with or entirely contradict results from similar studies. Other findings may demonstrate a rare consensus of opinion. Few scientists agree on the type of factors relating to back pain. Instead, much of the literature is structured in ways that inhibit meaningful comparison by emphasizing pathological conditions, personal qualities and risk factors common to back sufferers in that particular study, but oftentimes unrepresentative of broader occupational groups or populations. One of the most common methodological shortcomings is seen in the cross-sectional studies evaluating sedentary occupation and back pain. The reader should be aware that often, these studies do not take into account changes in jobs as a consequence of back trouble. Once the pain occurs, the worker may change to a less physically demanding job, lessening the apparent association between heavy manual work and back pain. For instance, one study found that 33% of office workers at a coal mine had previously worked as miners, yet the lifetime incidence of low back pain was greater among ex-miners in every age group than among those who had only worked in office jobs[12]. On the other hand, to the extent that employees overstate the amount of physical activity experienced on the job, bias would tend to make an association appear greater than it actually is.

Occupational Risk Factors

Heavy versus Sedentary Labor

Throughout industrialized societies, there is an emerging awareness of occupational disease as a cause of disability. It is being discovered medically and determined judicially that the spine can undergo injury at work without a specific accident occurring. The first recorded case of low back pain related to an occupation dates back to 2780 BC, when the Egyptian architect/physician Imhotep treating construction workers at the pyramid of Sakkara described a "sprain of a vertebra" in the spinal column[13]. While the succeeding centuries have witnessed an incredible transformation in the mechanization of the work place, the human spine remains as vulnerable to industrial risk factors as it has ever been. Manual material handlers represent the single largest group of industrial workers affected by back pain. Snook has found that more than half of all compensable back pain incidents are related to the manual handling of objects[14]. Lifting has been implicated in 37% to 49% of such cases; pushing in 9% to 16%; pulling, 6% to 9%; and carrying, in 5% to 8% of cases. Many of these occupations require the frequent movement of objects weighing 25 pounds or more, with a few requiring transport of material in excess of 100 pounds. Not surprisingly, it is the heavy industry sector of the economy that has been most vigorously researched for abnormally high back pain incidence and severity.

This section will explore a variety of different industries, each with unique physical requirements and environmental conditions. The occupations will include truck and bus driving, concrete reinforcement, construction, coal mining, steel, nursing, agriculture, paper, and various manufacturing jobs. Contrasted with these relatively stressful occupations, several reports will compare back pain incidence and severity among industrial workers with more sedentary careers – white-collar and service workers, computer programmers, housewives, and air traffic controllers.

Many studies have confirmed that workers in heavy industry are more likely to have low back pain[15-17]. Wickstrom found a higher prevalence of sciatica in concrete reinforcement workers than in computer technicians [18,19]. Hult showed the frequency of low-back pain was 52% in a group of 471 retail, light industry and sedentary workers, compared with a 64% incidence in 666 construction, food handling and other heavy industry workers [16,17]. The differences are less subtle than they appear, since the light industry workers had a 6.8% prevalence of severe back pain, compared to a statistically significantly 10.6% prevalence for the heavy industry laborers. Daniel reported that 71% of a low-back pain patient sample taken from a steel mill in North Wales were manual workers [20]. Of 100 employees chosen consecutively, only 19% had a history of low-back pain of less than six months, while 52% had suffered between six months and ten years, and 29% had a history of over ten years. Harley reported that 27% of individuals who developed pain were handling 50 pounds or more at the time of the injury [21].

Other investigators, however, have reported contradictory observations. Nachemsom, for example, has written that low-back pain occurs with the same frequency among sedentary workers and those doing heavy labor [22]. The finding by Wickstrom of increased incidence of sciatica among heavy laborers is by no means conclusive. Although the report documents a 40% rate of sciatica (pain radiating down the leg) and a 30% rate of lumbago (backache) among 295 Finnish workers, Wickstrom is careful to note that the "analysis did not bring forward any confirmation of the hypothesis that reinforcement work increases the incidence of low-back disorders. It is thus evident that the dose-response relationship between exposure to concrete reinforcement work and the appearance of back disorders, if it exists, is not strong enough not to be concealed by other factors."

Still, the evidence suggesting no difference in back trauma regardless of an occupation's physical demands is overwhelmingly contradicted by the majority of literature showing a linkage between back pain and heavy labor. Consider a 1984 study assessing the relationship between work environment and current and previous episodes of low-back pain by Damkot and Pope et al. [23]. A cross-section of several occupational groups consisting of 303 men was analyzed to determine which aspects of work history were most commonly associated with back pain. Participants were assigned to groups according to the intensity of back ailment: no pain, moderate pain, or severe pain. Among the 150 variables evaluated via questionnaire were activities such as standing and lifting, carrying, pushing and pulling, sitting, driving vehicles, and use of vibrating equipment. The age range was 18-55 for the three groups. 16% of the total were employed as manual laborers – carpenters, machine operators or mechanics – while 15.2% were involved in sedentary work such as administrative positions. The remaining 69% worked in both occupational sectors.

The authors believe a number of potentially significant findings emerge. No significant relationships were demonstrated between the three low back categories and the occupational categories, with the exception of truck driving. This exception is consistent with the data proposed by Kelsey who has concluded that truck drivers are four times more likely than the general population to have a disc herniation. As for body posture, 40% of the group without any low back pain, and 36% of the moderate low back pain group were required to stretch and reach during job performance, while 59% of the severe LBP group had such requirements. This finding is consistent with the highly publicized notion that workers engaged in heavy manual handling of objects held away from the body during lifting, bending, and twisting movements are more vulnerable to back injury than during any other job task [25,26]. The physical work demands for participants with low back pain were determined to be greater than the other groups. Also significant was the observation that occupational factors were only partially related to the severity of back symptoms, a testament to the complexity of back pain caused by a variety of both individual, environmental and psychological risk factors.

A clear distinction was identified between pain groups when asked if symptoms had occurred as a result of a specific, sudden event. Nearly 71% of the severe pain group said yes, compared with only 39% of the moderate pain group. The literature demonstrates that not all attacks of low back pain can be related to a particular accident or incident. Manning observed that 31% of 54 low-back injuries did not report any preceding accident with sudden onset of pain. In another study, a review of 500 low back patients by Rowe found that 65% of the cases had no associated accident [27,28]. Yet Buckle et al. observed 65% of a patient group to attribute the onset of back pain to a particular incident[29].

Afacan has noted a strong relationship between back stress, absenteeism and degree of physical labor experienced by coal miners [12]. It was found that 15% of the men (1795 out of 12,125 miners) were absent due to back pain, with the underground transport workers and coal face workers most vulnerable to frequent, prolonged absenteeism. Moreover, the underground workers were twice as likely as the surface workers to miss work, almost certainly caused by the constant stooping demanded by the low ceilings of the mine shafts. Undeutsch noted nearly identical risk factors above ground, among airport transport workers who frequently perform work using awkward positions in low, narrow spaces [30]. Of the 366 workers participating in the study, 66% reported current back symptoms during the last four weeks, while previous incidents of back pain were reported by 56%. Report of back pain correlated significantly with height, age, and length of transport work experience. For instance, 53% of the persons with a stature of less than 164 cm (5'5") demonstrated present back symptoms, compared to 73% of persons with a height over 178 cm (5'10").

In a similar report, Svensson and Andersson studied the relationship of low-back pain to work history and work environment in a randomized sample of 940 men, aged 40 to 47 [31]. Two main groups were structured to concentrate those who had experienced pain at some point in their lives and those with current symptoms or problems occurring at least once a month. The lifetime incidence of low-back pain in the sample was 61%, corresponding well to the results of previous studies, as demonstrated by Bergquist-Ullman and Biering-Sorensen [32,33]. The prevalence rate among those subjects experiencing monthly low-back pain was 31%. Sciatica was found in 40% of those with back trouble.

Several observations were noted in these studies. Back pain patients sat less at work than those without pain. This finding contrasts with the report by Magora who noted that individuals were equally likely to experience a higher incidence of back pain whether or not they stood or sat for any length of time, regardless of job type [34]. Svensson and Andersson also found heavy work to be strongly correlated with the occurrence of low-back pain, those performing the most grueling work having the highest incidence. An association between lifting and pain was also noted. Psychological factors were also important: men affected by low-back pain often had more monotonous work, demanding less concentration. In a different analysis using the same sample group from above, Svensson et al. was able to demonstrate several cardiovascular risk factors associated with low-back pain [35]. Angina pectoris, calf pain, breathlessness on exertion, smoking, physical activity at work and leisure, worry and tension, fatigue at the end of workday, and perception of stress were all positively correlated with lumbar pain. After covariate analysis, four independent variables were found directly related to pain: calf pain, smoking, high physical work activity, and frequent feeling of worry and tension.

And what of the epidemiological data regarding women and the occupational incidence of low-back pain? Nursing, for instance, has been identified by several investigators as a major cause of low-back pain in Finland, Britain, Sweden and the United States [36-39]. A review of worker's compensation claims in 26 U.S. states ranked nurses' aides in the top ten occupations for back injuries, alongside laborers and garbage collectors [40]. Magora et al. found that Israeli nurses reported a higher incidence of low-back pain than farmers, bus drivers and light industry workers [41]. Stubbs found that nurses have a high rate of recurring back pain, with 44% recalling at least seven episodes of back pain, compared with only 15% recalling only a single episode without recurrence [42]. Statistics from the Ontario Hospital Association report that among all hospital nursing personnel, back injury accounts for more than 40% of all time-lost claims [43]. Contrary to the popular misconception of nursing as a perfectly harmless occupation for dainty young ladies, the reality of the job requires some of the most physically demanding tasks of any occupation.

Most of the literature seems to implicate patient handling as the most common event triggering back pain, repeatedly supported in interview after interview with nursing personnel [37,40,44,45]. Dehlin et al. observed that 73% of nurses aides suffering from back symptoms considered patient lifting to be the heaviest task [39]. Another study attributed 38% of all back pain to patient handling incidents [42]. Based upon the following assessment of the occupational demands, it would appear that such activity has become an ergonomic nightmare: "Patients tend to be heavy, inefficiently shaped for lifting, and lack convenient handholds. Furthermore, they are unpredictable and may suddenly collapse or resist movement. Supportive lifting, pulling or pushing may be required on an irregular and sometimes emergency basis, when adequate assistance is not available. Close quarters, wide beds and inefficient work heights lead to awkward body postures and asymmetric forces" [46].

Videman et al. completed a study of 880 nurses to assess the primary risk factors contributing to spinal pathology [47]. Questionnaires were sent to 562 qualified nurses and 318 nurses' aides to clarify the prevalence of low-back pain associated with age, work-load, free time activities, menstruation, pregnancies and number of children. The two groups were distinguished by the fact that nurses' aides reporting a markedly higher number of hours per week devoted to lifting, bending and twisting, and the least time spent sitting as compared to qualified nurses.

Results indicated that 85% of the nursing aides and 79% of the qualified nurses had experienced low-back pain in the past, and the prevalence increased with age. Previous experience with sciatic pain was found in 38% of the qualified nurses and 43% of the nursing assistants, while the rates of previous back injury were recorded as 16% for the nursing assistants and 10% for the qualified nurses. Accordingly, acute musculoskeletal disorders as a cause of disability compensation increased with age, the risk for 25 year old nursing assistants being 3.4 times that of qualified nurses, and 4.5 times greater for developing sciatic symptoms. No differences of chronic disability were found between the two groups. Low back pain associated with menstruation, pregnancy and exercise was judged not statistically significant. It was concluded that for those under the age of thirty, the physical demands of work wer related to low-back pain in both groups of nurses. Perhaps the most interesting finding was the significant increase in pain of sciatic distribution with number of childbirths, primarily in the 25-34 and 45-54 age groups.

The same relationship between the intensity of the nursing task and susceptibility to back pain was noted in another study by Venning et al.[48]. During a year-long survey of 4306 nurses, 204 incidents of low back pain among 199 persons were observed, with the annual injury rate of the group calculated at 4.9%. Approximately 48% of the injuries did not require time away from work. Most importantly, four factors were determined by logistic regression to be significantly associated with the incidence of reported injury: job category, lifting, work activity, and previous history of reported back complaint. The statistics indicate that those nurses working in a service area where lifting occurs most frequently were nearly five time as likely to report injury than areas requiring the least amount of lifting. Similarly, daily lifters had an incidence rate 2.2 times that of the those lifting occasionally or not at all. In support of Videman's comparison of nursing assistants and qualified nurses, Venning observed the incidence for nursing aides to be 1.77 greater than for registered nurses and supervisory personnel, and 1.73 greater for individuals who had previously reported back injury, compared to those who had not reported previous injury. No other factors were significantly related to back pain, including age, physical activity, availability of lifting aids, height and weight and instruction in back care (despite the fact that 85% of all participants had received some form of instruction in general back care).

A more generalized study by Heliovaara examined the variable incidence of herniated lumbar disc or sciatica in 592 men and women during an 11 year period after an initial health examination [36]. For each incidence case, four control subjects matched individually for sex, age and place of residence were selected, with the age range of all participants between 20 and 59. Importantly, the "healthy worker effect" was avoided, a well-known problem in occupational epidemiology describing the tendency of ill people to switch to jobs not requiring full physical performance. The study was structured so that data on occupation and the physical demands of work referred to the time before symptoms in the back or leg developed.

Several professional and blue-collar occupations were analyzed, including forestry, agriculture, construction, chemical processing, manufacturing and transportation. Among the occupations employing women, housewives, white-collar and service workers, and agriculture were most common. The objective of the study was to identify the predictive power of various occupational factors causing hospitalization due to herniated lumbar intervertebral disc and/or sciatica. The results showed the incidence of pathology was smallest among men working in professional or other white-collar occupations, and highest among blue-collar workers in industry such as metal or machine workers. Motor vehicle drivers had the greatest risk of any occupation: risk of disc herniation was about three times that of professional workers, and risk of herniation or sciatica was over four times the lowest incidence rate.

The author found the occupational risks for women were clearly less variable than for men. Housewives appeared to have the lowest incidence of any group, while the mixed group of female industrial workers (not including occupations in the metal, paper or construction industry) showed the highest risk of being hospitalized because of disc herniation or sciatica. This rate was more than double the risk rate for female white-collar workers. One of the interesting conclusions was that self-assessed strenuousness of work did not predict herniated lumbar intervertebral discs or sciatica in men, whereas the women who had reported that they did light work showed a significantly lower risk than did women involved in normal or strenuous work. The moderate risk of herniation among male agricultural workers (mostly small-scale farmers) was also noteworthy, since farming is known to involve very heavy physical labor. This observation is completely at odds with the findings by Goodsell, who reported a particularly high incidence of lumbar herniation in farmers [49].

Additionally, Heliovaara is careful to note the limitations of the study: "Occupation and quality of work may have contributed either to herniation of intervertebral discs, to precipitating or aggravating symptoms of an old herniation, to proneness of the patient to seek surgery, to the clinical decision-making of physicians, or even to all of these events together.....Etiological appraisals must therefore be made with caution, and the present study cannot confirm, for example, the theory that occupationally induced stresses would damage lumbar intervertebral discs." (Figure 1-1)

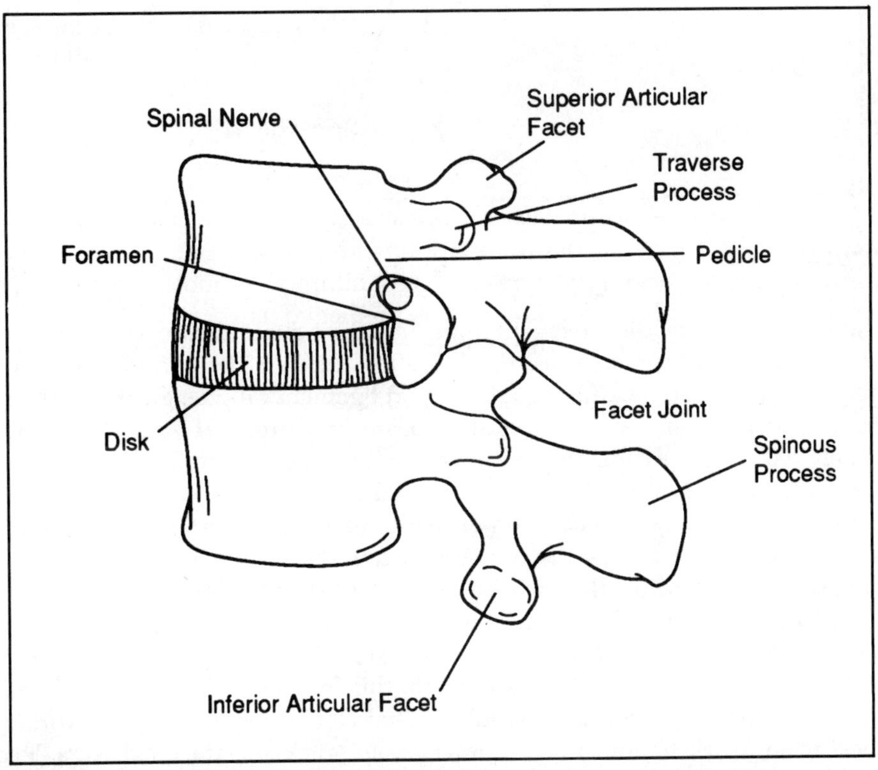

Fig. 1-1a.

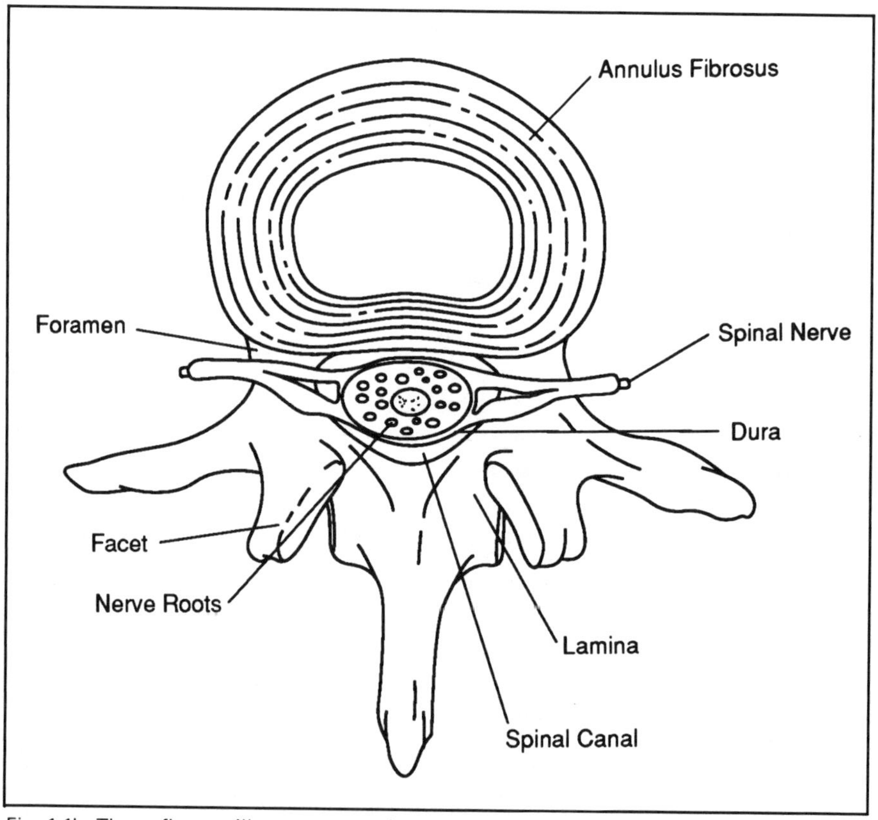

Fig. 1-1b. These figures illustrate some important anatomic features of the lumbar spine.

Vibration

The influences of vibration on the low back have received a great deal of attention, with little disagreement in the literature about the degenerative consequences of prolonged exposure. Vibration disrupts the natural movement frequency of the spine, causing muscle and ligament fatigue, greater vertebral creep, possible demineralization and spasm of peripheral vessels, and ultimately reducing the capability of the musculoskeletal system to safely manage load bearing. The most commonly reported effects of industrial vibration are low-back pain, early degeneration of the lumbar spinal system and herniated lumbar discs. Machinery that vibrates within the spine's 4.5-6 Hz frequency range is thought to do the greatest amount of damage, especially for those individuals who spend most of the day in a sitting position. A train, bus, motorcycle, tractor, bulldozer, jackhammer, backhoe, and motorboat are all examples of machinery that vibrate within this frequency range. Several studies have indicated abnormal musculoskeletal conditions in shipyard workers, sheet metal workers, miners, helicopter pilots, truck and tractor drivers, locomotive engineers and those using vibrational hand tools [50,51,52,53]. In fact, some reports suggest that the use of modern rotating and oscillating machinery may explain the lower incidence of low back pain in the lesser developed countries [54]. Many of these occupations such as pilot or driver appear to be quite harmless to the spine. While such workers rarely contend with handling heavy weights, the long-term exposure of the lumbar spine to vibration may be every bit as debilitating.

In an attempt to evaluate the effects of industrial vibration on the spine, Wilder, et al. designed an apparatus that replicated sinusoidal vibration [55]. Through the use of a hydraulic shaker powered by a 30-horsepower hydraulic pump, tests were carried out on 45 individuals, aged 18-39, with no prior history of low-back pain. Using an EMG to monitor the electrical activity of the spinal system, frequency sweeps were administered to each participant, who were then instructed to assume several common body postures, including extension, flexion and lateral bend.

Three peaks of enhanced transmissibility corresponding to the resonant frequency of the spinal system were found. The resonant frequencies are expressed as a ratio of input (measured from the seat of the apparatus) to output (measured by a head helmet). The greatest transmissibility of vibratory input occurred at the first resonant frequency (5Hz) where vibrational input passing through the spinal system caused marked enhancement of vibrational output. At the most active frequency, a ratio of 1.79 was calculated, meaning that for every 1 g of acceleration at the buttocks, 1.79 g was transmitted through the spinal system to the head. Hence, vibrational output was nearly double the initial input at this frequency, well within the 3-6Hz frequency range of the vehicles and machine tools noted earlier.

As for the effects of postural changes on vibrational transmission, all body postures except the forward flex position were found to decrease stiffness and transmission. The authors speculate that "symptoms of muscle insufficiency may occur because of the direct effects of the vibrations as well as the positional shifts as one attempts to avoid unfavorable vibrational postures." Interestingly enough, others have cited contradictory observations which demonstrate that such postural variations (increased flexion, axial rotation, and lateral bend) increase intradiscal pressure and increase EMG levels in the paraspinal muscles.

Vibration - Helicopter Pilots

To continue discussion of the insidious effects of vibratory-induced back pain, the reader's attention is directed to an occupation that is rather uncommon but nonetheless representative of several industries requiring long periods of sitting and exposure to constant vibration at the spinal resonant frequency. Because the two factors are found together in several occupations, there is a good deal of confusion in identifying the role that each factor plays in the development of back pain. While the pilot may appear to be well insulated from the seemingly harmless sounds of the whirling rotor blades or roar of the jet engines, the research that follows will indicate that these sounds, combined with the posture the pilot must assume during flight, are anything but trivial.

A preliminary study on back pain in helicopter pilots revealed an entirely different opinion on vibration than the preceding analysis. Shanahan et al. reported no statistical difference between two groups of pilots randomly assigned to either a vibration or nonvibration control group, in terms of time of onset of pain or intensity of pain [56]. As with the Wilder study, Shanahan designed an apparatus which could simulate environmental vibration experienced on the job. The objective was to investigate the two factors most widely implicated in the etiology of back pain among helicopter pilots -- vibration and posture. With reported prevalence rates of back pain among pilots exceeding 50% and a few reporting rates in excess of 75%, vibration seems like the obvious choice of responsible risk factor. Yet according to Shanahan, it is commonly accepted that the seating configuration in most helicopters force the pilot to bend forward in his seat and lean slightly to the left, almost certainly causing soft-tissue irritation [57].

The experiment involved the design of a seat and control stick closely conforming to the dimensions and specifications of a UH-1H helicopter. The seat was mounted to a Multi-Axis Vibration Simulator, programmed to reproduce vibration measured from the floor near the seat of a UH-1H in cruise flight. The frequency of the rotor blades at this speed was approximately 5.4Hz, close to the natural frequency range of the spine, as discussed earlier. Eleven subjects were selected, all of whom reported frequent back discomfort when flying the UH-1H for periods of less than two hours. Each participant was monitored for two separate two hour periods, one with vibration and one without. The periods were randomly assigned. During the test period, the subject simulated every action he would normally be expected to do to maintain flight. According to the Visual Analog Scale (VAS), pain intensity was uniformly described as a dull ache or numbness in the low back & buttocks without radiation in the legs. Perhaps the most significant finding was that simulated vibration had no meaningful influence on the time of onset or the intensity of pain reported by the participants. It was also observed that pain in most of the subjects was transient, generally lasting only a few hours after flight. According to the investigators, "the major etiologic factor in the rather stereotyped back pain reported by helicopter pilots is posture. Pilots are forced to assume a slumped and asymmetrical position for extended periods of time with little chance to change position."

Among the more informative findings is a German study by Fisher et al, who tested 221 helicopter pilots and 226 jet pilots [58]. A comparison of clinical and radiological data yielded a 61% prevalence rate of low-back pain in the helicopter group, versus 29% for the jet pilots. Helicopter pilots showed spondylotic changes of the spine much more frequently, especially those pilots logging more than 1500 hours of flight time. Unfortunately, this report does nothing to clarify the degree to which vibration or posture is implicated in the development of lumbar pathology. The same can be said for a survey of 145 air crew members (including pilots, flight engineers and air rescue medics) by Schulte-Wintrop et al.[59]. It was found that 40% complained of back pain while flying, 51% had pain after the flight, and 39% experienced back ache lasting for longer periods. Degenerative changes were observed in those airmen with the most severe chronic back pain. Differences were also detected in the body height of helicopter pilots during and after flight time, suggesting compression and narrowing of the intervertebral discs. Examining vibration and posture with the hypothesis that chronic stress is an etiologic factor in spondylolisthesis, Froom et al. compared the x-rays of 153 helicopter pilots versus 500 cadets and 109 transport pilots in an effort to demonstrate the variable incidence of spondylolisthesis [60]. Results indicated that helicopter pilots had four times the prevalence rate (4.5%) of cadets (1.0%) and transport pilots (0.9%). Froom concludes that vibrational forces may cause spondylolisthesis.

Vibration: Agriculture, Construction, Transportation

In addition to aircraft pilots, there are three other occupations that expose the spine to significant levels of vibration: agriculture (tractor drivers), construction work (earth moving equipment operators), and transportation (taxi, train, bus and truck drivers). Based on a point scale designed by Hulshof et al.[61] to rate the relative value of nineteen reports on occupational vibration, it was concluded that no single study reached an adequate score on all criteria (quality of exposure data, effect data, study design and methodology). Most studies failed to control for confounding variables, and only a few examined a control group. Despite these shortcomings, the following reports seem to provide convincing evidence that "long-term exposure to whole-body vibration is harmful to the spinal system."

Dupuis and Christ published a highly acclaimed longitudinal ten-year study of the incidence of back pain in tractor drivers [62]. Two-hundred eleven drivers entered into the study in 1961 and were followed until 1971, at which point only 106 participants still remained. Radiological examination clearly indicated dramatically increased degenerative changes. Spondylotic, osteochondrotic and arthritic conditions increased from 57% of all participants in 1966 to 80% in 1971, while reports of back ache increased 47% to 58% over the same period. Similar results were described by Hilfert et al. in a 1981 study which found periodic back pain in 70% of 352 earth moving construction operators, compared with 54% for an unexposed control group [63]. Based upon radiographic and physical examination, "degenerative processes of the lumbar vertebrae and intervertebral discs" (collectively defined as lumbar syndrome) was observed in 81% of the operators, versus 53% for the controls. A study of construction workers by Damlund confirms this finding, noting that more construction workers than controls working less physically demanding jobs were forced into early retirement because of low-back pain [64]. In the year before retirement, 68% of the construction workers had low-back pain, compared with 50% in the control group.

Several long-term studies of backache in the transportation industry have been reported. In a 1974 article by Gruber and Zipermann, 1448 male interstate bus drivers were compared with three control groups to assess spinal disorder [65]. The analysis focused on drivers with the most professional experience, emphasizing drivers in the 35-54 age group. The follow-up period ranged up to 22 years (1953-1974). Results indicated that experienced drivers had a higher prevalence of disc displacement, ankylosis of the spine, vertebrogenic pain syndrome and other spinal disorders, compared to the control group.

A significant correlation between prevalence rate and exposure level was demonstrated. It was postulated that the combined effects of working posture, off-balance movements in fatigued drivers and whole-body vibration may be the primary cause of these disorders. Gruber later completed a study of back pain in 3205 interstate truck drivers, comparing them to a control group of 1137 air traffic controllers (a group notorious for high levels of back pain) over a follow-up period of 25 years [66]. Prevalence rates were significantly higher for the truck drivers, compared to the controls and even the bus drivers noted in the previous study. There was a greater incidence rate of premature spinal degeneration and disc displacement. These results are consistent with the findings of Kelsey and Hardy, who calculated the increased risk of disc herniation to be 4.67 for truck drivers (most injuries occurring during manual loading and unloading of truck), and 2.75 for persons who spent half or more of their job-time driving [67].

Individual Risk Factors

The concept of middle-age as a predisposing cause of low-back pain brings the reader to the second section of epidemiological research discussed in this chapter. All of the studies mentioned thus far were concerned with the environmental factors and occupational hazards thought to contribute to low-back pain. This section will discuss some of the most widely reported individual risk factors associated with lumbar problems, including age, sex, height, weight, and physical fitness. Closely related to these variables are risk factors of a more anatomic nature. Musculoskeletal abnormalities like spondylolisthesis, spinal stenosis and scoliosis will not be included in this section, but will be addressed in the next chapter concerned with the etiology of low-back pain.

The Effects of Aging

As with other risk factors, there is no real consensus among the medical community on an association between age and incidence of back pain. Most researchers acknowledge that the age group between the fifth and sixth decade of life is most susceptible to backache. This frequently is the most productive time of life for the industrial worker. Others dispute the claim entirely. Intuitively, it would seem that with increasing age, a comparable progression of degeneration would occur, resulting in a higher probability of pain. Nachemson examined this logical relationship in a study of 195 subjects. An x-ray study of 40 year olds revealed that 72% had osteophyte formation and 24% showed disc space narrowing [68]. These rates dramatically increased for those in their 60s, reaching a 97% rate of osteophytes and a 60% incidence of disc narrowing.

The age-degeneration relationship is proven conclusively, but the numbers do not address the linkage of degeneration to back pain. Many investigators are quick to point out that patients without spinal or disc degeneration are just as likely to contract pain as those with pathology. These studies, involving large numbers of subjects, indicate that marked degeneration and other skeletal abnormalities do not necessarily indicate prior symptomatology. Additionally, it is argued that there is absolutely minimal association between abnormal x-ray findings and low-back pain. It is this degeneration-pain relationship that is at the heart of the controversy regarding age as a significant risk factor.

In the largest survey of back pain epidemiology ever reported in the United States (10,404 participants), Deyo and Tsui-Wu found that prevalence rises after the age 25 to a peak in the 55-64 year-old age range, with a falling prevalence after age 65 [69]. The prevalence trend for sciatic pain peaked earlier, in the 45-54 year-old range. The peak age of onset appeared to be 20-29 years, with few cases beginning before the age of 20 and the number of new cases declining after the third decade. The cumulative lifetime prevalence of low-back pain lasting at least two weeks was 13.8% Frymoyer agrees that men are less likely to experience low-back pain after the sixth decade, but reports that the incidence for women continues to rise[70]. Interestingly enough, the study by Deyo discovered particular racial and demographic differences that demonstrate a statistical correlation with low-back pain. Deyo reports that whites had a higher prevalence than blacks or other minority groups. The most remarkable difference appeared to be a race-sex interaction, between white males having the highest incidence of back pain (15%), and black males having the lowest (7.7%). The same investigation also discovered significant regional differences regarding epidemiology, finding the northeastern United States to have the lowest incidence of back pain and the highest prevalence in the western part of the country, with a rate nearly 38% higher than in the Northeast. Similarly, statistics from the U.S. Department of Health Education and Welfare found the rate of hospitalization for disk disease was 50% higher in the western part of the country than any other region [71]. One wonders if regional differences in the characteristics of clinical practice account for these statistics.

Another study suggests a 70% prevalence for all individuals between 40 and 60 years of age, based upon findings by Horal who estimated peak frequency of back pain to be in the fifth decade, while Hult, Lawrence and Hirsch estimated the peak to be in the sixth decade [7,10,15,72,73]. The study found the most usual time for back trouble to begin in the third decade. Accordingly, a combination of the figures results in the great majority of back pain taking place between the ages of 25 and 55. Magora found the incidence of low-back pain, absence from work and duration of symptoms to increase in linear relation to age [41,74].

Waddell argues exactly the opposite in his assessment of age as a predisposing factor for pain [75]. He states that "low back pain and disability does not progressively increase with age and does not correspond to age-related changes of disc degeneration." He supports his opinion with eight controlled studies and two reviews which show little relationship between clinical symptoms and radiologic changes of degeneration. Undeutsch found that the prevalence of both previous and present back symptoms increased significantly among individuals beyond the age of 45 [76]. Similarly, findings by Vallfors, Troup and Cairns have all demonstrated that age is a predictor of low-back pain [77-79]. In opposition to this viewpoint are the studies from Chaffin and Park and White, who like Waddell, have reported age to be of little significance [80-81].

Rather than age as a causitive risk factor of low back pain, Bigos et al. argues that the years of employment can be a more important variable, noting that low back symptoms among manual laborers often occur first within a few years of the beginning of employment [82]. The authors reported a significant inverse association between the incidence of back injury and duration of employment. It was found that in every age group, high-cost claimants were more common among workers with less than five years on the job compared to more experienced workers. Whether or not the onset of low back pain among these workers is related to lack of experience in handling heavy work loads, insufficient strength, or young age remains to be determined.

Anthropometry

Body height and weight as factors influencing the risk of disc herniaton are topics of spirited debate. Many studies have observed anthropometric measurements to be correlated with low back pain. For example, in a study of U.S. Army recruits during World War II, height and weight were identified as positively associated with herniated lumbar disc. Undeutsch found a significant positive correlation between the prevalence of back symptoms and height [76]. Added to the list are the studies of Gyntelberg and Hrubec, all of whom believe that "people who are prone to low back pain are, in general, taller than those who are not" [83,84]. But other studies found no relation between the prevalence of low-back pain and weight or height [83,27]. Brennan et al., for example, found no significant differences between two groups of subjects with and without herniated lumbar discs with respect to height, weight, strength, body composition or cardiovascular fitness level [5].

Height is implicated as a risk factor in a 1987 finding by Heliovaara [86]. Body measurements were analyzed for predictive value of lumbar disc herniation in 332 men and women previously hospitalized and positively diagnosed during an 11 year follow-up. Body height, thickness of triceps skinfold, and body mass index (weight/height) were investigated for their ability to predict hospitalization due to herniated lumbar disc. The results indicated body height to be a meaningful predictor of herniation in both men and women. On average, the relative risk based on height increased 5% in men and 4% in women for every centimeter (0.4 inches) in body height above 180 cm (5'11"). No statistically significant risk was found until height reached 180 cm in men and 170 cm (5'7") in women, at which point the risk of herniation in the tallest men and women were two and four times, respectively, that of their counterparts who were more than 10 cm (4") shorter. These results were not altered by body mass index, social class, or smoking. Neither the body mass index nor thickness of triceps skinfold proved to be significant in predicting herniation. Ironically, severe obesity appeared to carry less risk than moderately elevated body mass index.

Male versus Female: Sex-related Differences

Are men really more prone to low-back pain than women? That is the question which many studies have tried to address. Yet again there is a distinct polarity of opinion as described in the literature. A study by Cypress is representative of the muddled ambiguity concerning sex as a predisposing factor for back pain [87]. Data from the National Ambulatory Medical Care Surveys from 1977 and 1978 shows that males in the 45-64 age group had the highest rate of physician visits. Visit rates for men aged 15-64 were higher than those of women the same age. Perhaps, most importantly, men were considered more likely than women to have disc displacement, sprains, or strains of sacroiliac region and other unspecified parts of the back. Kelsey has verified in an earlier study that men were more prone to back pain arising from a heriniated lumbar disc [88].

For women, low-back pain etiology was more often the result of urinary tract diseases or osteoporosis. Although the severity of back pain was less serious for women than men, the author acknowledges that the difference between visits of men and women in which problems were rated as serious or very serious was not statistically significant. Others have suggested that women are more susceptible to back pain when exposed to heavy work. Magora accounts for a higher rate of low-back pain among women working in occupations requiring hard physical efforts -- much like the findings discussed earlier in the nursing studies [74]. The author concludes that differential diagnosis be considered before studying sex differences in complaints, suggesting the author remains undecided about the influences of sex as a risk factor.

Countering with a different opinion, Brown reports that the prevalence of low-back pain is higher among women than men [89]. In a general population study of a suburb of Copenhagen, Biering-Sornesen concluded that of the 449 men and 479 women examined and questioned, the men reached a peak frequency of low-back pain at the age of 40, while the women exhibited a steadily rising prevalence rate with increasing age: "It seems fair to conclude that low-back pain has a different natural course after the age of 50 -- women tend to have frequent or even accelerating symptoms, whereas men enter a quiet phase to the extent that they tend to forget the trouble they once had" [90].

In summation, most large studies have failed to demonstrate any clear-cut evidence that sex has a significant effect on the general frequency of back pain. Such conflicting results raise the issue of the degree to which particular social customs and economic factors influence the distribution of low-back pain between men and women.

Previous Incidence of Back Pain

Although back pain is characterized by a high spontaneous remission rate, it is also characterized by a high recurrence rate. One study noted recurrence in 90% of sick-listed patients, and 67% of symptomatic controls [10]. Biering-Sorenson's evaluation of the suburban Copenhagen population study emphasizes the prognostic value of previous low-back symptoms [90]. Regression analyses determined that a high frequency of low-back pain within the past year, a short interval since the last episode and an aggravated course of the pain since onset were all highly significant variables: "The more recently and frequently a person has had low-back trouble in earlier life, the more liable he or she will be to experience a new attack during the year to come" [10].

Steinberg argues that even for individuals who consult a physician, there is a 95% probability that back pain will occur within six months[7]. A prospective study by Troup found that 50% of those with back injuries were reinjured within one year [91]. Rowe found that 85% of low back patients had histories of intermittent episodes [27]. An analysis of 68 patients by Buckle et al. revealed that 27% were having their first attack of low-back pain, 41% had one to three previous attacks, and 28% presented a history of at least three prior episodes of back pain [92]. Previous incidence has also been cited by Chaffin and Park as a significant personal risk factor [93]. The same rates of recurrence (82-85%) have been observed in nursing personnel with back pain [48].

One of the drawbacks in considering prior history as a legitimate risk factor is uncertain recollection of the patient. A clear example of the problem is shown in the Copenhagen study by Biering-Sorensen who found that only 84% of a sample group gave the same answer to a question about ever having previous back pain when retested at an interval of 6 months [90]. Hence, the reliability of accurate recall limits the application of prior history in explaining current back problems.

Physical Fitness and Muscle Strength

Most investigators agree that 80% of all backaches are of muscular origin, while those caused by disc herniation are only 1-2% of all reported back problems. This section will briefly examine the effects of cardiovascular fitness, back and hamstring flexibility and abdominal muscle strength upon the incidence of lumbosacral pain.

A muscular system has three basic, highly essential, joint-related functions: stabilization of the joint, motor function, and protection of the joint. The major muscle groups contributing to back strength are the abdominal muscles, paraspinal muscles, and the pelvic girdle muscles. According to Frymoyer, "there is no doubt that reduced strength of flexor and extensor supportive musculature, tested under a variety of experimental conditions, are associated with chronic and often impairing low back pain" [94]. A 1979 study of 1,652 fire fighters by Cady revealed that those men with higher levels of fitness, emphasizing cardiovascular stamina, had an incidence of back injuries nine times lower than the least fit fire fighters [95]. Approximately 7% of the least fit group experienced low back pain, compared to 3% of the middle fitness group and less than 1% for the most fit group. A subsequent follow-up study reported that the introduction of cardiovascular fitness programs improved stamina, endurance, strength and flexibility [96]. As a result of increased cardiovascular fitness, even without significant increases in strength and flexibility, workers' compensation costs were reduced 25%.

An important methodological problem must be considered when interpreting data indicating an association between physical fitness and low-back pain. As will be discussed in the psychology section, there is great uncertainty whether or not this risk factor is a cause or effect of disability. The appropriate question an informed reader must ask is the following: Is poor abdominal and back muscle strength, reduced flexibility, and ligament resiliency and hamstring elasticity associated with a higher incidence of low-back pain, or is this the physical manifestation of back disease? Unfortunately, none of the studies we have analyzed to date have been able to conclusively rule out the possibility of muscle weakness stemming from back trauma. Until more data is reported on the effects of physical fitness in preventing back pain due to trauma, the legitimacy of this cause-effect relationship will remain an open question.

One of the few studies to investigate abdominal strength (weakness) as a variable factor contributing to low-back pain is the work of Suzuki et al.[97]. The analysis was based on a well-known (and controversial) theory that the abdominal cavity reduces the axial compression forces acting on the intervertebral discs when intra-abdominal pressure is raised by contraction of the abdominal muscles, reducing the demands upon the back muscles and ligaments [98,99]. Some have speculated that the curvature of the spine is directly related to the strength and tone of the trunk muscles, whereby hyperlordosis (excessive swayback) is associated with weak abdominal musculature, and vice-versa [100].

Ninety male patients with low back pain (with or without sciatica), between the ages of 20 and 39, were tested for the muscle strength and fatigability of the trunk flexors and extensors. The same procedure was used to test a control group of 50 adult males having no history of back pain. An isokinetic dynamometer was used to record strength at preselected controlled velocities transmitted through a lever arm attached to the body. The two groups were tested both isometrically and isokinetically. It was concluded that with regard to isometric contraction results, the control group displayed a significantly stronger trunk flexion capacity, with an average torque measurement of 87 joules (64 ft/lbs), versus only 70 joules (52 ft/lbs) for those with backache. Differences were also discovered in a trunk extension test, where the torque value for the group without back problems was 157 J (116 ft/lbs), compared with 134 J (99 ft/lbs) for the patients. The results indicate the "value of trunk flexor and extensor muscle strength in the controls to be higher than that in the patients with low-back pain... [as is] also true for the patients with low-back pain for less than one month." As for fatigue of the abdominals, results demonstrated that fatigue of the trunk muscles flexors was clearly greater in the patient group than in the controls, but no such relationship was demonstrated in the assessment of trunk extensors. Moreover, the authors determined the trunk flexors to fatigue more easily than the trunk extensors in both groups. Significantly, no statistical correlation of fatigability and duration of low-back disability was observed.

The study corresponds well with an earlier investigation by Alston et al.[101] who reported that patients with chronic low-back pain had generalized weakness of trunk muscle strength, hypothesizing that the weakness was due to disuse imposed by pain or fear of pain [101]. A 1984 finding by Biering-Sorenson supports this theory as well, demonstrating a lower isometric endurance of the back muscles, reduced flexibility and elasticity of the back and hamstring muscles, and greater anterior spinal hypermobility in a group of 449 men who had experienced low-back pain for the first time [102]. This observation suggests that back pain may be caused by excessive mobility, contributing to spondylolisthesis which has been linked to low-back pain. Mooney, however, claims "although individuals with back pain may become stiffer, certainly there is no reason to believe that hypermobility is related to the onset of back pain." [103]

Nachemson found an entirely different result, demonstrating no evidence to support the theory that back pain could be related to trunk muscle weakness [104]. A 1987 study by Mellin [105] evaluating the correlation between spinal mobility measurements with degrees of chronic low-back pain in 301 men and 175 women also contradicts the finding by Suzuki [105]. This very current report observed that lateral flexion and rotation had a stronger relationship with low-back pain than forward flexion and extension, those variables Suzuki attributes to backache. Additionally, it was found that thoraculumbar mobility had a higher correlation with low-back pain than mobility of the lumbar spine. Mellin concludes that "spinal mobility measurements, like physical measurements, have only moderate relationships with the degree of chronic low-back pain. However, spinal mobility measurements are useful for classifying patients and for planning and following their treatment."

The importance of muscle strength and physical fitness has also been evaluated by Yu and Rhot in a review of recent epidemiological literature [106]. Chaffin et al. suggested that workers with less muscle strength were more prone to low-back injury, calculating that the probability of a musculoskeletal disorder is up to three times greater when job lifting requirements approach or exceed the workers isometric strength capability [107]. (The reader is referred to the Prevention chapter for further information concerning pre-employment testing and placement). Neither Pederson et al. nor McNeil et al. found a relation between muscle strength (back or trunk muscles) and the prevalence of low-back pain [108,109]. Similarly, in an evaluation of pretreatment chronic back trouble in 151 men aged 54-63, Mellin indicated that trunk isometric extension and flexion strength had relatively low correlations with low back pain [110]. Yet Brown argued that prior development of postural fatigue was critical to future back problems because it rendered the back liable to subsequent injury [111]. Calliet agrees that muscle fitness is an important anatomical factor, since periodic muscle contraction must serve as an auxiliary stabilizer while the ligaments rest [112]. Limited resiliency in the ligaments, the primary stabilizer in preserving an upright posture, and poor muscle tone can cause an overload of the ligaments, ultimately resulting in back pain.

Pregnancy

Is childbirth related to the incidence of back symptoms? In a study of surgically proven herniated lumbar discs, O'Connell determined pregnancy to be a primary factor in back pain, arguing that "pregnancy is an etiological factor in the development of lumbar disc protrusion" [113]. King finds pregnancy related disc herniation to be a rare event [114]. It has been suggested that 50% of the pregnant patient population will experience some degree of low-back pain, with the incidence increasing with the number of pregnancies and age [115]. The primary etiology of pregnancy-related backache appears to be the sacroiliac joints, excessive lumbar lordosis, laxity of ligaments caused by the secretion of relaxin and possibly direct pressure of the fetus on the lumbosacral nerve roots [116,117].

For example, of 862 pregnant women interviewed in a recent Swedish study, about half reported some degree of low back pain [118]. Possibly one-third will experience severely disabling pain which could even interfere with walking. Sciatica in one or both legs will occur in one-half of this group. Another study by LaBan and Perrin conclusively demonstrated an extremely low incidence of pregnancy-induced disc herniation [119]. During a ten year period, an incidence of 1:10,000 was observed among a series of 48,760 consecutive deliveries, with only five pregnant patients reporting herniated lumbar disc symptoms. Of possible significance, each patient was delivered by caesarean section. The author states that "although the mechanical and postural stresses of pregnancy have been cited as predisposing causes of a herniated lumbar disc, this study suggests otherwise." However, both LaBan and Kelsey agree that pregnancy which terminates in normal delivery predisposes subsequently to herniated lumbar disc disease [119,120].

Fast et al. interviewed 200 women within one to two days after giving birth and found that 56% of the group suffered from low-back pain during pregnancy [121]. Of particular interest is the racial distribution of pain among the patients, with Caucasians reporting significantly more pain than Hispanics (34% versus 15%). Further analysis demonstrated that the age, weight gained by the mother during pregnancy, baby's birth weight, number of prior pregnancies, and number of prior children were not related to back pain.

Smoking

It now seems that spinal disorders can be added to the long list of diseases associated with cigarette smoking. While the mechanisms for this association is not entirely clear, several theories have been proposed. Frequent coughing has been observed to cause increased intradiscal pressure. Another plausible explanation concerns the positive correlation between smoking and diminished bone mineral content. Microfracture of the intervertebral end-plates caused by osteoporosis can result, thus inhibiting the flow of nutrients into the disc and rendering it more susceptible to mechanical deformities. Reduced discal metabolism and end-plate microfracture could also result from reduced blood flow to the vertebral body, as seen in dogs injected with the nicotine equivalent of one cigarette. Other variables that explain why smoking is a risk factor include the high probability that such individuals do not exercise regularly (if at all), and the alleged link between heavy smoking and anxiety or depression. Both of these variables are somewhat predictive of low back pain.

The empirical evidence supporting these views is quite convincing. For instance, Frymoyer evaluated the percentage of smokers among 3920 persons aged 18 to 55 with and without low back pain [122]. The low back pain sufferers were more likely to be cigarette smokers, particularly when smoking was accompanied by a chronic cough. It was found that while 13.6% of subjects did not report back pain, nearly three times (33%) as many smokers did experience pain. For women, 12.1% of the participants without back pain smoked, but more than twice as many smokers (26%) reported pain. Cox et al. observed nearly identical statistics in a study of 576 low back or leg pain patients, noting smokers among 33% of low back/leg pain sufferers, as compared to 14% of those without pain [123]. Additionally, it was found that those with no pain tended to be nonsmokers who exercised more frequently for longer periods of time than pain patients. Kelsey et al. found cigarette smoking to be associated with an increased risk for prolapsed disc, increasing 20% for each 10 cigarettes smoked per day during the past year [124]. Another study by Svensson et al. also demonstrated a higher incidence of back pain among smokers than among non-smokers [125].

Psychosocial Risk Factors

Much of the epidemiological research surveyed thus far demonstrates that pain has an important subjective component, and that there is no clear relationship between the amount of tissue damage and the degree of discomfort reported. It has long been recognized that certain psychological elements and social variables related to the occupational environment influence the way in which the individual perceives back pain. Yet by the same token, many believe pain to be a contributing factor to the manifestation of psychological and social instability. The literature is divided on whether back pain is accompanied by a greater incidence of psychological strain, or whether that same psychosocial instability results in an increased susceptability to back trouble. Unfortunately, a conclusive answer remains elusive. The very subjectiveness of back pain prohibits any meaningful isolation of the factors involved in reported pain, making it impossible to assign any cause or effect relationship.

Rather than argue over the chronology and basis of the linkages, the remainder of this section will sift through a variety of studies and analyze those psychosocial-pain relationships which have been observed in industry. The following articles will provide some compelling evidence demonstrating that the incidence of low-back pain can be evaluated in terms of the social and psychological stability of the individual. Variables including the degree of emotional distress, neuroticism, job satisfaction, job security, level of education, and social isolation will be discussed in terms of their association with increased incidence and intensity of low-back pain.

A report by Vallfors investigated the disputed link between these factors and back pain [78]. Two hundred-twenty participants, taken from the ranks of both blue-collar and white-collar occupations, were divided into two groups -- one group with objective evidence of pathology, the other with no evidence of objective pathology, presenting with normal mobility and musculature, a negative straight-leg-raise and no signs of neurologic involvement. The two groups were then classified, according to the duration of symptoms: subacute (0-3 months with slow onset), acute (0-3 months with immediate onset), and chronic (minimum of 3 months). The study considered the history of each patient ten years prior to treatment and one year after treatment.

This study demonstrated that 51% of the patients were unable to present objective evidence of back pain, even though all participants claimed injury. This figure included 40% of the acute group, 34% of the subacute, and 70% of the chronic patients. Furthermore, the proportion of patients without objective findings increased with increased duration of absenteeism and duration of pain, as did psychological and social problems. Of the chronic cases lacking any objective evidence of pathology, 68% presented with at least three of Waddell's five non-organic signs: superficial tenderness, a simulation test evaluating the rotational capability of the patient without the patient's awareness, distraction, regional or sensory weakness, and overreaction. None of the patients with objective findings displayed even one positive Waddell sign. It was also found that 80% of the patients without objective findings were manual laborers. On the other hand, 67% of the patients with objective findings were manual laborers.

More important were the factors proven to be statistically significant in relation to back pain among the non-objective group. Those patients were more frequently unmarried and divorced, especially manual workers in the acute and subacute groups. In addition, the worker's housing environment was generally worse and their wives or husbands often worked outside the home. These non-objective cases were also dissatisfied with their work mates, and had greater frequency of neurosis, migraine, ulcer and smoking habits. Significant differences in alcohol consumption were also revealed. Thirty-one percent of the chronic patients without objective findings demonstrated signs of alcoholism, compared with only 2% for the patients with objective findings, or with patients with subacute/acute back conditions. The level of education was significantly lower for all three groups (acute, subacute and chronic) when compared with the control group.

Vallfors concludes: "If the job is subordinated, monotonous and physically and psychologically strenuous, then the risk for absence due to low-back pain increases. Social factors play an equally important role, particularly in those where more than 50% of the back patients have no detectable objective symptoms can be detected . . . Social, psychosomatic, psychological, alcoholic problems, dissatisfaction with their work mates, working conditions and working environment all seem to force the patients to report themselves ill... The question then arises as to whether these patients should be considered low-back patients at all!"

Unlike the Vallfors report, a cross-sectional study of a Swedish pulp and paper company found the incidence of back pain was related more directly to the physical aspects of the work place rather than accompanying psychological aspects [126]. Eastrand evaluated psychosocial factors associated with back abnormalities and self-reported back pain. A questionaire was given to each of the 391 male participants, assessing school and training, working conditions, family relations, housing conditions, house keeping, social contacts, leisure activities, financial status, health, and for the oldest age group, a question regarding attitudes toward retirement. Only 42% of the participants suffering from back pain presented objective signs of abnormality. Surprisingly, the association with neuroticism (based upon the Marke-Nyman test) was stronger for organic pain than for pain lacking physical origin. This finding contradicts the view that neuroticism is associated with non-organic back pain, as Vallfors asserts.

Additionally, the psychosocial work-related factors just listed did not show any significant association with back pain or back abnormality. However, it was observed that back pain, and especially back abnormality was associated with low income, low education and occupational status. Not surprisingly, this association is strongest for manual workers, suggesting an inverse relationship between education level and job strenuousness. Recognizing the unusually disproportionate differences in back pain and/or abnormality between clerks and manual workers from the plant, it would appear that it is the physical factors in the work environment that are the most important determinants of back disorder. Others have also found social factors to be of little significance. An evaluation of the predictive factors associated with return to work after rehabilitation failed to denote any statistically relevant social factor in an analysis of 52 chronic low-back patients [127]. Marital status, family environment, welfare office registration, income, smoking and alcoholic habits were all observed to have no prognostic value whatsoever.

Schaepe approaches the risk category in a different way, proposing a direct relationship between the incidence of low back pain and the degree of job security, work stimulation, freedom of movement and the degree of input of abilities and education [128]. The proposed theory, endorsed by Nerrell, asserts that the psychosocial environment derived from the work organization and structure contributes to fear of injury, monotony and anxiety, all of which cause stress [129]. According to Nerrell, it has been determined that when psychosocial work stress is present, nervous tension and consequent muscle tension lead to an over-use of muscles not actually needed for the job, causing increased fatigue and greater probability of injury. In fact, the incidence of low-back pain was calculated to be twice as frequent in workers suffering from psychological work stress than in those able to cope.

Similar results were seen in a group of 21 men between the ages of 50 and 59, selected from both blue and white collar industries. The subjects were interviewed in an attempt by Hultman to identify "the healthy back person" [130]. The participants were asked questions pertaining to education, profession, mechanical and mental stress during present and previous work, leisure activities, life conditions, health status and heredity concerning low back trouble. The most statistically significant finding was that 20 out of 21 participants experienced a high degree of independence in the work place, and 17 stated their jobs to be very satisfactory.

In a series of individual studies from 1970-1975, Magora evaluated the physical, psychological and socioeconomic demands encountered in eight different industrial occupations [131-137]. Those participants with low back pain felt their jobs were more physically demanding, were less satisfied with their occupation and social status, and described their jobs as requiring greater mental concentration and responsibility than the control group. It was concluded that the worker's subjective assessment of an occupation's physical demands and greater overall mental and physical responsibilities can also affect the incidence of low back pain.

A much larger sample from Dayton, Ohio was evaluated to compare sociodemographic factors related to self-reported low back pain among a random population, based on the study variables of age, gender, occupation, physical demand of occupation, income, education and marital status [138]. Of the 2792 subjects participating in the study, frequent back pain was reported by 499 persons, a prevalence of 18% well within the 15% to 20% annual incidence range of back pain which much of the literature accepts. It was found that prevalence of back pain is generally greater for persons no longer married than for those who are married. More specifically, the results of a multivariate analysis indicated a steep increase in prevalence coming with increasing age among persons who are no longer married, a very small increase associated with age among married persons, and a sharp decrease in back pain prevalence related to increasing education among married individuals.

In this large sample, the highest significant incidence rate was observed among those between 50 and 64 years of age who were no longer married, regardless of educational level. An expected prevalence rate of 44% to 46% was calculated for women, and 40% to 42% for men. This contrasts markedly with the lowest expected prevalence rate for those 50-64 year olds who were married and had completed more than a high school education, men demonstrating a 9% rate and women a 13% incidence rate. In fact, within the same age/education group, those persons no longer married had three times the incidence rate.

It is theorized that those individuals no longer married must "contend with decreased social supports and increased responsibility in all areas of daily living. This may lead to physical and emotional stress, which in turn may precipitate or aggravate back pain". The negative association between reported back pain and education level is thought to be a result of the high probability that persons with greater education are more likely to take jobs in the professional and managerial occupations that are not as physically demanding. Others have added to the explanation by recognizing the stress and anxiety many blue-collar workers must feel when their livelihood depends largely upon health, possibly resulting in premature return-to-work before a back injury has healed, thereby causing reinjury and chronic symptoms [139,140].

One report indicates that educational level can be the most significant risk factor of any discussed thus far, and probably one of the very few factors that does not change over time, as it is nearly always established before the onset of low-back pain. Using data from the National Center for Health Statistics considered to be a representative sample of the entire United States civilian population, Deyo and Tsui-Wu evaluated the correlation of socioeconomic factors with back pain in 1516 individuals [141]. Compared with a control group who had never experienced back pain longer than two weeks duration, those reporting back pain were significantly older, less educated, less likely to have been working for most of the prior year and had much less income.

The single most important result of this study was the importance of education level as a prognostic factor for back pain. It was discovered that for men, education level was more directly related to back disability than self-rated pain severity, age or income. According to Deyo, educational level has such a strong predictive power because it encapsulates many other variables relating to job satisfaction, degree of job strenuousness, overall health and medical treatment: "Educational level may influence the 'attractiveness' of one's work, and thus, motivation to return to full activities. Some have suggested that persons with greater education are better able to understand health risks and to alter their behavior accordingly; furthermore, they may use medical care more effectively. Education level is also associated with altered preferences regarding job risk and lower cigarette consumption... and is strongly associated with health status in the general population."

As the preceding studies have clearly demonstrated, marriage and education are only two of many variables which relate to the psychological and social environment of the low-back sufferer. Such factors in and of themselves do not predispose an individual to back trouble; it is the linkage between the variable and consequent emotional and muscular stress that will influence the perception of back pain, even if back pain is without organic origin. Indeed, many of the individual and occupational risk factors discussed in the prior sections of this chapter, which one might reasonably associate with back pain, may have no effect at all because certain psychosocial conditions diminish the perception of back pain.

For example, one might logically expect that with increasing age comes a similar increase in reported pain. While it is true that age brings on progressive degeneration which has been linked to pathology, it should never be assumed that the individual will automatically experience symptoms. In fact, Mechanic et al. discovered that in a sample population of 937 subjects, exactly the opposite was true [142]. A linear relationship was demonstrated whereby increasing age was associated with decreasing reports of back pain, even though the older respondents were considerably more likely to show objective evidence of pathology.

A detailed analysis provided some very intriguing statistics. It was found that those participants aged 56 or older were more than two times as likely to display physical findings than the 25-45 age group, and three times as likely to have five or more such findings. Yet in contrast to this data, those aged 65 or older were least likely to complain, while those in the 46-55 age group were most likely to complain. The relationship was still proven statistically significant even after rigorous multivariate and regression analysis. An assessment of the mental condition of the participants was also given, revealing that those with depressed moods were more than twice as likely to demonstrate physical findings, and complained more often than those with a more positive outlook.

The discrepancy between objective evidence of back pain and subjective complaints can be readily understood when one considers the common belief that pain perceptions are dependent upon psychological context and social comparison. It is hypothesized that rather than consider elderly persons to be healthy optimists, "a more viable suggestion is that the elderly adjust their perceptions because of modified health expectations with age.... It is plausible to anticipate that assessments of pain are shaped by context, what people expect of themselves, and the consequences of pain for the roles and tasks they must assume.... they are more likely to normalize bodily discomforts."

Summary

In an effort to present a current, precise and objective overview, throughout this book the reader will be struck by the variability and contradictions inherent in this study of low back pain. Respected researchers disagree about whether or not heavy work increases the incidence of low back pain. Some authors argue that all job types are equally likely to produce lumbago and sciatica while others make convincing arguments that truck driving, helicopter piloting, and nursing pose significant risks for a worker's back.

Does increasing age result in increasing back pain? Many factual articles conclude that maturity is associated with back pain while others indicate that pain decreases with time. Increasing height has been shown to correlate with increasing back problems by some authors but not by others. Some see men as greater back pain sufferers, while others find women more susceptible.

Strong muscles and high levels of general fitness are often touted by researchers as keys to reducing the severity and frequency of back pain. Other students of the subject remain unconvinced and see no value in exercise. Even among those who advocate muscle conditioning there are arguments about which muscles to work on and how strong they need to be.

Few authors dismiss psychological factors as important in the overall back pain picture. Defining just which factors are significant has not been easy, however. Low education seems to correlate with low back pain problems. Perhaps drug and alcohol abuse does too. The overall picture is not yet clear, but an effort must be made to present what information is currently available.

References

1. Mayer TG, Gatchel RJ, Mayer H, Kishino ND, Keeley J, Mooney V: A prospective two--year study of functional restoration in industrial low back injury -- An objective assessment procedure. JAMA 258:1763, 1987.
2. Report of the Panel on Pain to National Advisory Neurological and Communicative Disorder and Stroke Council. NIH Publication No. 81:1912, 1979.
3. Caruso LA, Chan DE: Evaluation and management of the patient with acute back pain. The American Journal of Occupational Therapy 40(5):347-351, 1986.
4. Yu T, Roht LH, Wise RA, Kilian J, Weir FW: Low back pain in industry — An old problem revisited. J. of Occup Med. 26 (7):517-522. July 1984.
5. Caruso LA, Chan DE: Evaluation and management of the patient with acute back pain. The American Journal of Occupational Therapy 40(5):347-351, 1986.

6. Sandstrom J: Clinical and social factors in rehabilitation of patients with chronic low back pain. Scand J Rehab Med 18:35-43, 1986.
7. Steinberg, GS. The Epidemiology of Low Back Pain. Low Back Pain, edited by Stanton-Hicks M, Boas R. New York: Raven Press, 1982, pp 1- 12.
8. National Safety Council: Accident Facts, 1973-1981.
9. Dillane JB, Fry J, and Kalton G. Acute back syndrome – a study from general practice. Br. Med. J., 3:82-84, 1966.
10. Horal J. The clinical appearance of low back disorders in the City of Gothenburg, Sweden. Acta Orthop Scand (Suppl), 118: 8-73, 1969.
11. Brena SF, Turk DC: Vocational disability: A challenge to pain rehabilitation programs. In Aronoff GM: Pain centers in the US: A revolution in health care. New York, Raven Press, 1988.
12. Afacan AS: Sickness absence due to back lesions in coal miners. J Soc Occup Med 32:26-31, 1982.
13. Brandt-Rauf PW, Brandt-Rauf SI: History of occupational medicine: relevance of Imhotep and Edwin Smith papyrus. Br J Indust Med 44:68, 1987.
14. Snook SH, Campanelli RA, Ford RJ: A study of three preventive approaches to low back injury. J Occup Med 20:478, 1978.
15. Magora A: Investigation of the relation between low-back pain and occupation: Age, sex, community, education and other factors. Ind Med Surg 39:465-471, 1970.
16. Hult L: The Munkfors investigation. Acta Orthop Scand Suppl 16:76, 1954.
17. Hult L: Cervical, dorsal and lumbar spinal syndromes. Acta Orthop Scand (Suppl) 17:102, 1954.
18. Wickstrom G, Hanninen K, Lehtinen M, et al: Previous back syndromes and present back symptoms in concrete reinforcement workers. Scand J Work Environ Health 4 (suppl 1):20-28, 1978.
19. Wickstrom G, Nummi J, Nurminen M: Restriction and pain during forward bending concrete reinforcement workers. Scand J Work Environ Health 4(suppl 1):29-38, 1978.
20. Daniel JW, Fairbank JCT, Vale PT, et al: Low-back pain in the steel industry -- A clinical, economic and occupational analysis at a North Wales integrated steel works of the British Steel Corporation. J Soc Occup Med 30:49-56, 1980.
21. Harley WJ: Lost time back injuries -- their relationship to heavy work and pre-employment back x-rays. J Occup Med 14:611-614, 1972.
22. Nachemson AL: Low back pain, its etiology and treatment. Clin Med 78:18-24, 1971.

23. Damkot DK, Pope MH, Lord J, Frymoyer JW. The relationship between work history, work environment and low-back pain in men. Spine 9 (4): 395-399, 1984.
24. Kelsey JL: An epidemiological study of acute herniated lumbar intervertebral discs. Rheum Rehab 14:144-159, 1975.
25. Andersson GBJ: Epidemiological aspects of low back pain in industry. Spine 6:53, 1981.
26. Kelsey JL, Githens PB, White AA, III, et al: An epidemiologic study of lifting and twisting on the job and risk for acute prolapsed lumbar intervertebral disc. J Orthop Research 2:61, 1984.
27. Manning DP: Slipping accidents causing low-back pain in a gearbox factory. Spine 6:70-72, 1981.
28. Rowe ML: Low-back pain in industry -- a position paper. J Occup Med 11:161-169, 1969.
29. Buckle PW, Kember PA, Wood AD, et al: Factors influencing occupational back pain in Bedfordshire. Spine 5:254-258, 1980.
30. Undeutsch K, Gartner KH, Luopajarvi T, Kupper R, Karnoven MJ, et al: Back complaints and findings in transport workers performing physcially heavy work. Scand J Work Environ Health 8(suppl):92-96, 1982.
31. Svensson HO, Andersson GBJ: Low-back pain in 40 to 47 year-old men: Work history and work environment factors. Spine 3:272-276, 1983.
32. Bergquist-Ullman M, Larsson U: Acute low-back pain in industry. Acta Orthop Scand (Suppl) 170:1-117, 1977.
33. Biering-Sorensen F: Low back disorders - a community problem. Paper presented at Odense Hospital, Denmark. Oct 5, 1979.
34. Magora A: Investigation of the relation between low-back pain and occupation. III. Physical requirements. Sitting, standing and weight lifting. Industr Med Surg 41:5-9, 1972.
35. Svensson HO, Vedin A, Wilhelmsson C, Andersson GBJ: Low-back pain in relation to other diseases and cardiovascular risk factors. Spine 3:277-85, 1983.
36. Heliovaara: Occupation and risk of herniated lumbar intervertebral disc or sciatica leading to hospitalization. J Chron Dis 3:259-264, 1987.
37. Cust G, Pearson JCG, Mair A: The prevalence of low back pain in nurses. Int Nursing Rev 19:169-179, 1972.
38. Dehlin O, Hedenrud B, Horal J: Back symptoms in nursing aides in a geriatric hospital: an interview study with special reference to the incidence of back symptoms. Scand J Rehabil Med 8:47-53, 1976.
39. Dehlin O, Berg S, Hedenrud B, Andersson G, Grimby G: Muscle training, psychological perception of work and low-back symptoms in nursing aides. Scand J Rehabil Med 10:201-209, 1978.

40. Klein BP, Jensen RC, Sanderson LN: Assessment of workers' compensation claims for back strains/pains. J Occup Med 26(6):443-448, 1984.
41. Magora A, Taustein I: An investigation of the problem of sick-leave in the patient suffering from low-back pain. Ind Med 38(11):80-90, 1969.
42. Stubbs DA, Buckle MP, Hudsons PM, et al: Back pain in the nursing profession. I. Epidemiology and pilot methodology. Ergonomics 26:755-765, 1983.
43. Workman's Compensation Board Annual Report. Toronto, Ontario Workman's Compensation Board, 1980, 1981, 1982.
44. Bigos SJ, Spengler DM, Martin NA, et al: Back injuries in industry: A retrospective study. II. Injury factors. Spine 3:252-256, 1986.
45. Harber P, Billet E, Gutowski M, et al: Occupational low-back pain in hospital nurses. J Occup Med 27(7):518-524, 1985.
46. Agnew J: Back pain in hospital workers. Occup Med 3:609-616, 1987.
47. VidemanT, Nurminen T, Tola S, Kuorinka I, Vaharanta H, Troup JDG: Low-back pain in nurses and some loading factors at work. Spine 9(4):400-404, 1984.
48. Venning PJ, Walter SD, Stitt LW: Personal and job-related factors as determinants of incidence of back injuries among nursing personnel. J of Occup Med 29(10):820-825, 1987.
49. Goodsell JO: Correlation of ruptured lumbar disk with occupation. Clin Orthop 50:225-229, 1967.
50. Cossu F: Cervical spondylosis in workers using vibrating instruments. Nunt Radiol 33:308-312, 1967.
51. Fahrni WH: Conservative treatment of lumbar disc degeneration: Our primary responsibility. Orthop Clin North Am 6:92-103, 1975.
52. Fusco M: Effect of vibration on the peripheral vascular system and on the vertebral column. Folia Med 46:361-372, 1963.
53. Rosegger R, Rosseger S: Health effects of tractor driving. J Agric Eng Res 5:241-276, 1960.
54. Andersson GBJ, Ortengren R, Schultz A: Analysis and measurement of the loads on the lumbar spine during work at a table. J Biomech 13:513-530, 1980.
55. Wilder DG, Woodworth BB, Frymoyer JW, Pope MH: Vibration and the human spine. Spine 3:243-254, 1982.
56. Shanahan DF, Reading TE: Helicopter Pilot Back Pain -- A preliminary study. Aviat Space Environ Med 55 (2):117-21, 1984.
57. Sliosberg MR: A propos des douleurs vertebrales du pilote d'helicopteres: Consequences therapeutiques et prophylactiques en jonction de leur etiologie. Rev Med Aeron 2:263-268, 1962.
58. Fisher V, Witt AN, Troger O, Troger H, Beck A: Vibrationsbedingte wirbelsauleschaden bei hubschrauberpiloten. Arbeitsmed Sozialmed Praventivmed 15:161-163, 1980.

59. Schulte-Wintrop HC, Knoche H: Backache in UH-1d helicopter crews. AGARD-CP 255(19):1-12, 1978.
60. Froom P, Froom J, Dijk D van, Caine Y, Ribak J, Margaliot S, Floman Y: Lytic spondylolisthesis in helicopter pilots. Aviat Space Environ Med 55:556-557, 1984.
61. Hulshof C, van Zanten BV: Whole-body vibration and low-back pain -- A review of epidemiologic studies. Int Arch Occup Environ Health 59:205-220, 1987.
62. Dupuis H, Christ W: Untersuchung der Moglichkeit von Gesundheitsschadigungen im Bereich der Wirbelsaule bei Schlepperfahrern. Heft A. Max-Planck-Institut fur Landarbeit and Landtechik, Bad Kreuznach, 1972.
63. Hilfert R, Kohne G, Toussaint R, Zerlett G: Probleme der Ganzkorperschwingungsbelastung von Erdbaumaschingenfuhrern. Zentralbl Arbeitsmed 31:199-206, 1981.
64. Damlund M: Low-back pain and early retirement among Danish semiskilled construction workers. Scand J Work Environ Health 8(suppl 1):100-104, 1982.
65. Gruber GJ, Zipermann H: Relationship between whole body vibration and morbidity patterns among motor coach operators. NIOSH, 1974.
66. Gruber GJ: Relationships between whole body vibration and morbidity patterns among interstate truck drivers. NIOSH, 1977.
67. Kelsey JL, Hardy RL: Driving of motor vehicles as a risk factor for acute herniated lumbar intervertebral disc. Am J Epidemiol 102:63-73, 1975.
68. Nachemson A; from Steinmann M: The American Medical Association Book of Back Care. Random House, 1982.
69. Deyo RA, Tsui-Wu YJ: Descriptive epidemiology of low-back pain and its related medical care in the United States. Spine 3:268, 1987.
70. Frymoyer JW, Cats-Baril W: Predictors of low-back pain disability. Clin Orthop 221:89-98, 1987.
71. Vital and Health Statistics: Utilization of short-stay hospitals, Annual Summary of the United States, Series 13-Number 41, 1977. U.S. Dept. of Health, Education and Welfare, Washington D.C.
72. Lawrence, JS: Disc degeneration -- its frequency and relationship to symptoms. Ann Rheum Dis 28:121-136, 1969.
73. Hirsch C, Jonsson B, Lewin T: Low-back symptoms in a Swedish female population. Clin Orthop 63:171-176, 1969.
74. Magora A: Investigation of the relation between low-back pain and occupation. I. Age, sex community, education, and other factors. Ind Med Surg 39:465-471, 1970.
75. Waddell G: A new clinical model for the treatment of low-back pain. Spine 7:644, 1987.

76. Undeutsch K: Back complaints and findings in transport workers performing physically heavy work. Scand J Work Environ Health 8(suppl 1):92-96, 1982.
77. Vallfors B: Acute, subacute and chronic low back pain, clinical symptoms, absenteeism and working environment . Scan J Rehabil Med 11:1-98, 1985.
78. Troup JDG: Straight-leg-raising and the qualifying tests for increased root tension: Their predictive value after back and sciatic pain. Spine 6:526, 1981.
79. Cairns D, Mooney V, Crane P: Spinal pain rehabilitation: Inpatient and outpatient treatment results and development of predictors of outcome. Spine 9:91, 1984.
80. Chaffin DB, Park KS: A longitudnal study of low-back pain as associated with occupational weight lifting factors. Am Ind Hyg Assoc J 34:513-525, 1973.
81. White AWM: Low back pain in men receiving workmen's compensation. Can Med Assoc J 95:50, 1966.
82. Bigos SJ, Spengler DM, Martin NA, et al: Back injuries in industry: A retrospective study. III. Employee-related factors. Spine 11:252, 1986.
83. Gyntelberg F: One year incidence of low back pain among male residents of Copehagen aged 40-59. Dan Med Bull 21:30-36, 1974.
84. Hrubec Z, Nashold BS: Epidemiology of lumbar disc lesions in the military in World War II. Am J Epidemiol 102:366-376, 1975.
85. Brennan GP, Ruhling RO, Hood RS, Shultz BB, Johnson SC, Andrews BC: Physical characteristics of patients with herniated intervertebral lumbar discs. Spine 12(7):699-702, 1987.
86. Heliovaara M: Body height, obesity, and risk of herniated lumbar intervertebral disc. Spine 5:469-471, 1987.
87. Cypress BK: Characteristics of physician visits for back symptoms: A national perspective. Am J Public Health 4:389-395, 1983.
88. Kelsey JL: An epidemiological study of acute herniated lubar intervertebral discs. Rheumatol Rehabil 14:144-153, 1975.
89. Brown JR: Factors contributing to the development of low-back pain in industrial workers. Am Ind Hyg Assoc J 36:26-31, 1975.
90. Biering-Sorenson F: A one-year prospective study of low back trouble in a general population -- The prognostic value of low back history and physical measurements. Danish Med Bull 5:362-375, 1984.
91. Troup JDG, Martin JW, Lloyd DCEF: Back pain in industry: A prospective survey. Spine 1:61-69, 1981.
92. Buckle PW, Kember PA, Wood Ad, et al: Factors influencing occupational back pain in Bedfordshire. Spine 5:254-258, 1980.

93. Chaffin DB, Park KS: A longitudnal study of low back pain as associated with occupational weight lifting factors. Am Ind Hgy Assoc J 34:513-525, 1973.
94. Frymoyer JW: Predictors of low-back pain disability. Clin Orthop 221:89-98, 1987.
95. Cady LD, Bischoff DP, O'Connell ER, Thomas PC, Allan JH: Strength and fitness and subsequent back injuries in fire fighters. J of Occup Med 21:269-272, 1979.
96. Cady LD, Thomas PC, Karwasky RJ: Prgogram for increasing health and physical fitness of fire fighters. J Occup Med 27:110, 1985.
97. Suzuki N, Endo S: A quantitative study of trunk muscle strength and fatigability in the low-back pain syndrome. Spine 1:69-74, 1983.
98. Bartelink DL: The role of abdominal pressure in relieving the pressure on the lumbar intervertebral discs. J Bone Joint Surg 39B:718-725, 1957.
99. Morris JM, Lucas DB, Bresler B: Role of the trunk instability of the spine. J Bone Joint Surg 43A:327-351, 1961.
100. Asmussen E, Heeboll-Nielsen K: Posture, mobilty and strength of the back in boys 7 to 16 years old. Acta Orthop Scand 28:174-189, 1959.
101. Alston W, Carlson KE, Feldman DJ, Grimm Z, Gerontinos E: A quantitative study of muscle factors in the chronic low back syndrome. J Am Geriat Soc 14:1041-1047, 1966.
102. Biering-Sorensen F: A one-year propsective study of low back trouble in a general population. Dan Med Bull 31(5):362-375, 1984.
103. Mooney V: Where is the pain coming from? Spine 12(8):754-759, 1987.
104. Nachemson A, Lindh M: Measurement of abdominal and back muscle strength with and without low back pain. Scand J Rehabil Med 1:60-65, 1969.
105. Mellin G: Correlations of spinal mobility with degree of chronic low back pain after correction for age and anthropometric factors. Spine 5:464-468, 1987.
106. Yu T, Roht LH, Wise RA, Kilian DJ, Weir FW: Low-back pain in industry -- an old problem revisited. J of Occup Med 7:517-524, 1984.
107. Chaffin DB, Herrin GD, Keyserling WM: Pre-employment strength testing -- an updated position. J Ocup Med 20:403-408, 1978.
108. Pederson OF, Petersen R, Staffeldt ES: Back pain and isometric back muscle strength of workers in a Danish factory. Scand J Rehabil Med 7:125-128, 1975.
109. McNeil T, Warwick D, Andersson G, Schultz A: Trunk strengths in attempted flexion, extension, and lateral bending in healthy subjects and patients with low-back disorders. Spine 5:529-538, 1980.
110. Mellin G: Chronic low back pain in men 54-63 years of age. Correlations of physical measurements with the degree of trouble and progress after treatment. Spine 11(5):421-426, 1986.

111. Brown JR: Lifting as an industrial hazard. Am Ind Hyg Assoc J 34:292-297, 1973.
112. Calliet R. Low Back Pain Syndrome. FA Davis, Philadelphia, 1982.
113. O'Connell JEA: Lumbar disc protrusions of pregnancy. J Neurol Neurosurg Psychiatry 23:138-141, 1960.
114. King AB: Neurologic conditions occurring as complications of pregnancy. Arch Neurol Psychiatry 63:611-644, 1950.
115. Mantle MJ, Greenwood RM, Currey HLF: Backache in pregnancy. Rheumatol Rehabil 16:95-101, 1977.
116. Epstein JA: Treatment of low back pain and sciatic syndromes during pregnancy. NY State J Med 59:1757-1768, 1959.
117. Sands RX: Backache and pregnancy: Method of treatment. Obstet Gynecol 12:670-676, 1958.
118. Berg G, Hammar M, Moller-Nielsen J, Linden U, Thorblad J: Low back pain during pregnancy. Obstetrics and Gynecology 71(1):71-75, 1988.
119. LaBan MM, Perrin JCS, Latimer FR: Pregnancy and the herniated lumbar disc. ArchPhys Med Rehabil 64:319-321, 1983.
120. Kelsey JL, Greenberg RA, Hardy RJ, Johnson MF: Pregnancy and the syndrome of herniated lumbar intervertebral disc: An epidemiological study. Yale J Biol Med 48:361-368, 1975.
121. Fast A, Shapiro D, Ducommun EJ, Friedman LW, Bouklas T, Floman Y: Low back pain in pregnancy. Spine 12(4):368-370, 1987.
122. Frymoyer JW, Pope MH, Constanza MC, et al: Epidemiologic studies of low back pain. Spine 5:419, 1980.
123. Cox JM, Trier KK: Exercise and smoking in patients with and without low back and leg pain. J of Manip and Physiol Therap 10(5):239-245, 1987.
124. Kelsey J, Githens P, O'Conner T, Ulrich W, Calogero J, Holford T, et al: Acute prolapsed lumbar intervertebral disc. An epidemiologic study with special reference to driving automobiles and cigarette smoking. Spine 9:608-613, 1984.
125. Svensson H: Low back pain in relation to other diseases and cardiovascular risk factors. Spine 8:277-285, 1983.
126. Eastrand N: Medical, psychological, and social factors associated with back abnormalities and self reported back pain: A cross sectional study of male employees in a Swedish pulp and paper industry. Br J of Ind Med 44:327-336, 1987.
127. Sandstrom J: Clinical and social factors in rehabilitation of patients with chronic low back pain. Scand J Rehab Med 18:35-43, 1986.
128. Schaepe JL: An occupational perspective. In Stanton-Hicks M, Boas R (eds.): CHRONIC LBP. Raven Press, 1982.

129. Nerell G, Waghlund I: Stress factors in the working environments of white collar workers. From: Reducing Occupational Stress. Dept. of Health, Education and Welfare. (NIOSH). No. 78-140, pp. 62-72.
130. Hultman G: The healthy back, its environment and characteristics: a pilot study. Ergonomics 2:295-298, 1987.
131. Magora A: Investigation of the relation between low back pain and occupation. Part I. Ind Med 39(11):31-37, 1970.
132. Magora A: Investigation of the relation between low back pain and occupation. Part II. Ind Med 39(12)28-34, 1970.
133. Magora A: Investigation of the relation between low back pain and occupation. Part III. Ind Med 41(12)5-9, 1972.
134. Magora A: Investigation of the relation between low back pain and occupation. Part IV. Scand J Rehabil Med 5:186-190, 1973.
135. Magora A: Investigation of the relation between low back pain and occupation. Part V. Scand J Rehabil Med 5:191-196, 1973.
136. Magora A: Investigation of the relation between low back pain and occupation. Part VI. Scand J Rehabil Med 6:81-88, 1974.
137. Magora A: Investigation of the relation between low back pain and occupation. Part VII. Scand J Rehabil Med 7:141-151, 1975.
138. Reisbord L, Greenland S: Factors associated with self-reported back pain prevalence: A population-based study. J Chron Dis 8:691-702, 1985.
139. Haber LD: Disabling effects of chronic disease and impairment. II: Functional capacity limitations. J Chron Dis 26:127-151, 1973.
140. Hirschfield AH, Behan RC: The accident process I. Etiological considerations of industrial injuries. JAMA 3:193-199, 1963.
141. Deyo RA, Tsui-Wu Y: Functional disability due to back pain. A population-based study indicating the importance of socioeconomic factors. Arthr and Rheum 30:1247-1253, 1987.
142. Mechanic D, Angel RJ: Some factors associated with the report and evaluation of back pain. J of Health and Soc Behavior 28:131-139, 1987.

CHAPTER 2

Etiology of Back Pain

Introduction

Despite the overwhelming volume of research and diagnostic technological advances providing state-of-the-art imaging, the ability of the physician to determine the cause of low back pain has not improved in several decades. Even though accounts of lumbago and sciatica are described in the Bible and in the writings of Hippocrates, a reasonable and scientific explanation for the etiology of low-back pain did not emerge until 1934 with the publication of the classic paper by Mixter and Barr on the pathology of disc herniation and nerve root pressure [1]. Nachemson summarizes the enigma with remarkable insight: "Having been engaged in research in this field for nearly 25 years and having been clinically engaged in back problems for nearly the same period of time, and as a member and scientific advisor to several international back associations, I can only state that for the majority of our patients, the true cause of low-back pain is unknown" [2].

In this age of nuclear magnetic resonance imaging and computed axial tomography, why does one of the world's most distinguished back scholars acknowledge that the etiology of the lumbar pain remains an unsolved mystery? Back pain, it will be recalled, is a symptom and not a disease. Low back pain should be considered as a final common pathway, a complaint for a number of different disease states. It can even be an indicator of malignancies, visceral diseases or vascular problems. Such etiological ambiguity is a direct reflection of the complex anatomy of the spine — an intersection of many pain-producing soft tissues, including the articular joints and corresponding innervation, anterior/posterior ligaments, the ligament flavum, the periosteum, quadratus laborum muscles, fascia and of course, the bundles of branching nerve fibers which pass along the spinal canal and through the foraminal openings of each vertebra.

As a result of this anatomical complexity and the concentrated proximity of these tissues, the etiology of back pain remains largely unknown in most cases. Several studies have noted that as few as 15% of all patients can be given a specific cause of pain, while the remainder are idiopathic in nature. Dillane et al. reported the specific cause of low back pain was unknown in 79% of the men and 89% of the women experiencing their first episode of pain [3]. Lawrence writes of his experience in the UK, reporting that the most frequent diagnosis was disc degeneration, which accounted for 12% of a population sample x-rayed for spinal pathology [4]. Osteo-arthritis of the lumbar facet joints was found in 5% of the patients, sacro-iliac joint disease in 2%, rheumatoid arthritis in 3%, while nerve root pressure from disc prolapse or other sources was found in less than 10% of the subjects. The remaining 65% of the cases had non-specific back pain, ascribable to unknown causes.

Over the last twenty years there has been an explosion in the terminology used to describe the causes of low-back pain, including lumbosacral strain, lumbar disc disease, sciatica, lumbago, spondylosis, spondylolysis, spondylolisthesis, osteoarthritis, spinal stenosis, myofascial pain syndrome, sacroiliac sprain, myalgia, fibrositis, degenerative disc disease, internal disc disruption, and other musculoskeletal verbiage. The symptom of spondylosis alone has been defined as degenerative arthritis, hypertrophic arthritis, discogenic disc disease and osteoarthropathy [5]. All of the above are symptoms linked to pain, some of which are reported to account for 50% to 90% of all diagnoses [6].

The value of such highly descriptive terminology is at best debatable, and at worst, utterly confusing to both the patient, administrator, and medical researcher interested in evaluating diagnostic information. As an example of how this affects the patient, a survey of 490 subjects was undertaken to evaluate the diagnosis and treatment of low-back pain [7]. Over 50% of these patients received two or more different diagnoses from two or more practitioners. The most common etiology diagnosed by orthopedic surgeons (visited by 429 patients) was low back syndrome. Those visiting chiropractors (422 patients) were most likely to hear an etiology of "misalignment," followed by "subluxation, twisted pelvis, spinal curvature, pinched nerves and malformed hips." Only 10% of all participants received the same diagnosis from two or more practitioners, and even those seeing practitioners in the same field resulted in a paltry 29% concurrence rate. The author was careful to highlight in large capitals the fact that no other major area of medical diagnosis has a worse track record.

The etiology of lumbar spinal pain can be divided into three distinct categories, according to assumed pathology. Degenerative and traumatic disease is probably the most commonly attributed causal factor, and includes intervertebral disc herniation, spondylolysis, spondylolisthesis and osteoarthritis. A second category includes structural abnormalities: scoliosis, spinal bifida occulta, hyperlordosis, kyphosis, as well as other congenital spina deformities. The third etiological category concerns muscular and ligamentous dysfunctions. All will be discussed in terms of the biomechanical and biochemical processes contributing to lumbar pathology.

This chapter will try to organize the gamut of back abnormalities listed above into these three primary pathological conditions. In maintaining our objective format, dozens of studies will be cited to support or contradict a given explanation of low-back pain. The research will draw upon a significant amount of material concerned with the anatomy of the spine, as it is impossible to appreciate the logic of any proposed theory without an understanding of the function and composition of the underlying muscles, ligaments, bones and nerves.

Degenerative And Traumatic Disease

Spondylosis, Disc Degeneration and Herniation

Most of the medical community accepts the fact that the chronology of degeneration has a biomechanical and biochemical explanation. The literature cannot agree about the sequence of degeneration, but many believe the deterioration of the intervertebral disc is the primary culprit in the breakdown of the the spinal unit mechanism. What follows is a generally accepted evolution of spondylosis, defined as the degeneration of the disc possibly resulting in approximation of the posterior joints, synovial and capsular thickening, degeneration of articular cartilage, adhesions, osteochondral fractures, and even lose body formation.

Indicative of the pervasive and inevitable influences of disc degeneration seen world-wide, consider the results of an experiment in which a Swedish population was x-rayed for signs of vertebral deterioration. It was found that of those in their fifth decade, 72% presented with osteophytes, while 24% presented with narrow discs. By the seventh decade, 97% had osteophytes and 60% demonstrated disc narrowing [8]. Rowe found that 70% of 500 Kodak employees with back pain followed for 20 years had symptoms referable to degenerative disc disease [9]. The sequence included increments of minor annular damage beginning after age 25, advancing through the stage of gradual herniation of nuclear material in the 30 to 40 age group. The process continued to include intervertebral instability with narrowing of the neural foramina. This was followed by subluxation of the facet joints in the forties with further degenerative arthritis of the facet joints and marginal spur formation by the late forties and early fifties. The degenerative process concluded with scar formation and loss of mobility at the involved intervertebral segment in the middle to late fifties.

Puschel claimed that by the age of 20, the disc had reached maximum development and degenerative changes henceforth became the norm [10]. Lawrence reports that 60% of males and 44% of females over the age of 35 show definite osteophyte formation and narrowing, rising to 81% and 79% respectively by the age of 75 [4]. In a study of over 4000 spines, Schmorl and Junghanns agree, finding degenerative changes present in 50% of the population (4353 spines analyzed) by the age of 50, in 70% by the age of 60, and in 90% by the age of 70 [11].

It would it seem, therefore, that disc degeneration is a natural occurrence for everyone, although Fahrni has demonstrated the condition to be a rarity in non-industrialized societies [12].

Our description of the chronology of disc degeneration begins with a change in the capability of the disc to metabolize nutrients. As a result of improper disc nutrition the disc begins to dehydrate. Lewinnek has indicated that the relative amount of water in the disc decreases from 87% to 70% while the proportion of collagen increases, perhaps as a result of a failure to maintain an adequate cellular metabolism [13]. As the disc loses water and other nutrients, it begins to lose its original shape, shrinking in height and bulging out along the sides, causing the longitudnal ligament to slacken and pull away from the vertebral body, leading to excessive loads on other support structure.

Yet others dispute the association of disc thinning with disc degeneration, arguing that disc bulge "like an underinflated automobile tire" is a misleading analogy of degeneration that is atypical of elderly spines. Contrary to popular belief, Twomey and Taylor assert that average disc height is maintained or increased in a normal population of elderly persons [14]. In their opinion, the most significant factor in age-related changes of the lumbar disc is a weakening of the vertebral end-plates. Results from a measurement study of 204 cadaveric lumbar spines could not confirm a loss in disc height, but rather, significant increases in disc height with aging in L2-3, L4-5, and L5-S1 for both sexes.

The most revealing measurement was the significant decline in bone density with increasing age in both sexes, caused by the inevitable development of osteopenia/osteoporosis. It is strongly suspected that the loss of bone density leads to a reduction in the number of horizontal and vertical trabeculae, the system of reinforcing ties or cross-braces that help preserve the rigidity and structure of vertebral bone. Ultimately, fracture of the trabeculae causes end plate microfracture, as the adjacent disc expands into the concave upper and lower end plates of the vertebra. In some extreme cases, the disc has been known to herniate through the cartilaginous end-plate into the cancellous bone of the vertebral body, causing the formation of Schmorl's nodes. Depending on the the degree of structural damage, disc nutrition can be radically diminished as the nutrients are no longer able to diffuse freely through the end-plate, leading to disc dehydration. While it seems pointless to debate whether the end plate or the disc itself is responsible for variation in disc height and thickness associated with degeneration, it is critically important to acknowledge the fact that regardless of the specific pathogenesis, any alteration of the disc-end plate interface induced by a "ballooning" disc and end-plate concavity will cause an approximation of the vertebral bodies, and probably contribute to the dysfunction of other adjacent tissues.

With disc dehydration also comes a consequent loss of elasticity in the annulus fibrosus. The annular fibers undergo concentric tearing and radial fissuring, in some cases causing segments of the annulus to break off as free-floating fragments. Because of the normal lumbar lordosis, this degeneration falls mainly in the posterior lateral area, at the site where it is least reinforced by the posterior longitudnal ligament. At this point, the disc is increasingly prone to damage as it is less able to absorb or contain the stresses between the vertebra. Sudden strains, particularly if associated with rotational torque, could cause tearing and ultimate rupture of the annular wall. Gradual deterioration of the annulus fibrosus is the more common occurrence, the product of cumulative stresses over time, causing microscopic tears rather than a single explosive rupture. Interestingly enough, compressive force in a healthy disc will generally fracture the vertebral body before tearing the annulus. This is important when considering the relationships of traumatic events such as auto accidents or injuries at work to a herniated disc which may manifests itself several years later.

Surprisingly, little or no pain may be felt by the patient during this degenerative process until the disc material swells outward with increased annular fissuring and begins to irritate the nerve fibers of the outer annulus. Contact with a nerve root, or a structure containing nerve fibers (like a ligament) will be a source of sharper pain. Up until this point, degeneration of the annular fibers will not be a source of pain because neither nerve endings nor nerve fibers have been observed within the disc. In less than 20% of patients with weakening or tearing of the annulus, a large fragment of disc material will protrude through the opening, producing the infamous herniated disc [15]. In most cases, complete rupture does not occur. The annulus becomes more incompetent and weaker, but never completely loses its integrity.

Once nuclear material begins to protrude from the disk, or if there is significant disc bulging, several pain-producing structures are brought into play. The periosteum, the dura mater, the facet joint capsule, the dorsal surface of the ligamentum flavum, the interspinous, anterior and posterior ligaments, and the lumbodorsal fascia are all richly innervated, and all are potential sources of pain [13]. For instance, the ligamentum flavum shortens secondary to narrowing of the disc and subluxation of the facet joint. The elastic ligament then thickens and is passively pushed into the neural space [16]. This corresponds to Calliet's account of the "Multifidous Triangle," which extends from L4 to the iliac crest and down to the sacrum [5]. The area contains many pain-producing soft tissues, including the facet joints, the transversus ligament and the quadratus lumborum muscles.

As the vertebral end plates degenerate, sclerotic changes may result. As a consequence of osteophytes and settling, the foramen begins to narrow. Encroachment of any anatomical part into the spinal canal results in at least some stenosis. Brown notes that in an extreme situation, there may be a massive nuclear protrusion in which a large volume of disc material is suddenly thrust into the spinal canal, producing a "profound neurologic catastrophe" such as cauda equina syndrome [16]. A herniation of this type can cause disturbance of bowel and/or bladder functions, including total urinary retention, loss of sphincter reflexes, progressive motor weakness, and even paralysis.

Fortunately, this scenario is rare. Generally, the extrusion is a gradual and intermittent process, characterized by progressive foramenal narrowing, causing compression and inflammation of the nerve root. The end result is local pain and/or sciatica, depending upon which nerve roots are affected. Another product of disc narrowing is subluxation of the facet joints, causing a restriction of mobility. Simultaneously, degenerative changes on the cartilaginous surface of the facet joints can cause osteoarthritic local pain. We now have the three immediate by-products of this chronology of degeneration: spinal stenosis, nerve root entrapment, and osteoarthritis.

The degree of compression of either the spinal cord or the nerve root may well determine the course of a number of more serious, potentially debilitating conditions, such as pseudo claudication and cauda equina syndrome. Not only is the size of the herniation important, but also the direction of the herniation and the shape of the spinal canal. Many individuals, for example, can present evidence of a large disc herniation, yet never experience disability or even pain because of the large diameter of their spinal canals, which prevent compression of pain-producing tissues and nerves. Whether or not the disc herniates to the side of the dural sac (posterolateral being the most common direction) or towards the middle it may also determine the difference between mild and debilitating pain. In cases of cauda equina syndrome, etiology is nearly always due to a large medial disc herniation which compresses several nerve caudal nerve roots. Medial compression can cause perianal numbness, loss of anal reflexes, and disruption of the lower abdominal organs.

There are those that question the validity of associating disc herniation with disc degeneration. O'Connell suggests that herniation occurs at an earlier age than disc degeneration [17]. It was demonstrated in 500 cases requiring surgery that 4% of the group were between the ages of 11-20, 35% were 21-30, 38% were 31-40, 18% were 41-50 and 5% were between 51-60. Consequently, the author proposes that nuclear prolapse rarely occurs in the terminal fibrotic stages of disc herniation. Brown concludes that herniation is a much greater threat in the individual between the ages of 30 and 50, having good turgor in the nucleus, than in the elderly, in whom the nucleus is dessicated and fibrotic [16]. Consistent with this observation is a study by Weber which found that incidents of back pain among a sample population generally occurred during the morning hours of the day, when the increased hydration of the nucleus pulposus (turgor) is at its maximum [18]. The research of Adams and Hutton also supports the claim, offering evidence that disc herniation was significantly easier to produce in well-hydrated, healthy discs, whereas the older degenerative discs were relatively resistant [19]. It was concluded that "herniations therefore tend not to occur in degenerated discs."

Calliet concludes by emphasizing the viscious circle of degeneration: "When a disc degenerates, the extruded material allows further vertebral approximation, further ligamentous slackness, more dissection of the ligamentous-periosteal attachment, and thus further protrusion of nuclear material to fill the void. Disc compression keeps forcing material outward, constantly pressuring the posterior longitudnal ligament." Nachemson adds: "Without doubt the mechanical integrity of the intervertebral disc proper influences all the surrounding structures. When the disc degenerates there is an increase in facet load, altered distribution of stress concentrations in the end plates and subchondral bone of the vertebrae, encroachment on the nerve root canal and an increased demand for the muscles, especially the intersegmental groups, to stabilize the motion segment" [20].

The pathogenesis of disc degeneration just described is merely a model that suggests which elements of the back might be a source of pain, why they became a site of pain, and how they might affect other adjacent or distant parts of the body. The top priority of this section is to assess the linkage between objective evidence of intervertebral disc degeneration and low-back pain. As the reader will discover, the association between these variables is quite controversial.

Lawrence evaluated the relationship between pain and stages of disc degeneration, using a grading system from the Atlas of Standard Radiographs of Arthritis to measure the degree of degeneration [4]. Grade 1 is doubtful, presenting ambiguous evidence of osteophyte formation on the vertebral lip. Grade 2 is minimal, having a more definite osteophyte buildup, while Grade 3 contains marked osteophyte formation and disc narrowing. In Grade 4, the disc space has almost disappeared. The study documents a 4% incidence of sciatica with neurological signs of nerve root pressure in a group of 710 participants with grade 0-1 disc degeneration, 6% with grade 2 (minimal disease), and 10% with grade 3-4. The author concludes: "Those with Grade 3 and 4 disc degeneration are more likely to have nerve root pressure but this is only a small proportion of those with local or referred pain in the segmental distribution of the degenerate disc."

In a different study that analyzed the effects of injection of contrast material into a series of discs, there was a strong correlation between the amount of solution injected and exact reproduction of pain [21]. Using the same technique of disc injection, Hirsch et al. obtained the same results using saline solution[22]. The solution was also injected near the facet joint, causing pain in the back, the sacroiliac joint region, the gluteal area, and inferolaterally to the region of the greater trochanter. However, injection into the spinous ligament, the supraspinous ligament, and the ligamentum flavum caused only mild local irritation. The implication of these findings is that the gradual symmetric (non-traumatic) aging process is not painful but the nonsymmetric disruptive process is persistently painful, probably due to abnormal nutrition caused by asymmetry.

One finding that lends support to the theory of a disc degeneration-back pain relationship is a survey by Sachs et al, who discovered that only 3% of painful discs could be considered to be radiographically normal, as determined by CT scan discogram [23]. Unfortunately, this was one of the very few studies that demonstrated such a clear cut relationship. In separate studies Horal, Hult, and Hussar and Guller all found the incidence of degenerative changes in a low-back pain population to be no higher than in a control group of healthy subjects, as seen in the x-rays [24-26]. Significantly, these three early investigations did not utilize the newer imaging modalities currently available. Flor et al. agrees that "none of the well controlled studies found any relationship between radiologically documented changes of the spine and low back pain" [27]. Nachemson is also a disbeliever: "There are no consistent radiological findings associated with injury of the back that can lead one to the etiological cause of back pain." [28]

Earlier we mentioned vibration as a major occupational risk factor in the incidence of lumbar pain. Sandoval gives an insightful review of prior research which evaluated the connection between vibration and lumbar pain, emphasizing the importance of disc nutrition via the end-plates of the vertebra [29]. Several cited studies (Nachemson, Rolander & Blair) hypothesized that since the nucleus pulposus can only absorb nutrients osmotically through either the annular wall or the vertebral end-plates, the loss of permeability in either membrane would restrict the needed fluids from entering the nucleus [30,31]. Furthermore, it was suggested that the natural aging process, chemical change or mechanical damage could inhibit the function of the end-plates.

What about the effects of vibration? It has been documented that dynamic loading (i.e. vibration) has resulted in microfractures of the end-plate and trabeculae [32-35]. Based upon this evidence, Sandoval proposes that the vibration-induced microfractures of the end-plate and/or subchondral trabeculae lead to a reduced area for nutrient diffusion, which is the same conclusion discussed above by Twomey [14]. Moreover, the weakened annulus becomes increasingly vulnerable to dynamic shear, bending or rotational loading, causing an acceleration of degeneration and possibly disc herniation. A professional driver, for instance, regularly experiences several hours of road shock that may not be significant enough to cause injury by itself, but the postural and muscular components inter-related with vibration will add stress to the spine. If the driver is subjected to a barrage of such shocks, by the end of the day when his spine has been conditioned by the sum total of static, vibratory and muscular stress up to that moment, susceptibility to injury may be increased [14]. One does not have to have a specific incident occur in order to sustain injury.

It will be remembered that posture may also be a significant component in low-back pain, as demonstrated by various reports on helicopter pilots and other transportation professionals. Besides neural compression, disc nutrition is probably the most obvious etiological explanation of the anatomical mechanics of degenerative pain. In a discussion of the effects of posture on the diffusion of nutrients into the the lumbar discs, Adams and Hutton demonstrate that postural variation influences the fluid flow of the nutrient supply [36]. Specifically, it was observed that postures involving lumbar flexion (especially the sitting position) caused a larger outflow of fluid from the disc than did erect postures. This outflow is reversed when the spine is unloaded at night. The interaction of biomechanical and biochemical factors is thus implicated in the degeneration of the intervertebral disc.

The most significant aspect of the report was the conclusion that since erect, lordotic posture constantly reduces nutritional diffusion of the compressed posterior disc in favor of the anterior half of the disc, a flexed posture (sitting, for example) reverses the nutritional outflow by reducing the thickness of the posterior annulus by an average of 37%, thereby allowing less osmotic resistance and more effective penetration of nutrients. The authors conclude: "There can be little doubt that lumbar disc nutrition is improved by alternating flexed postures with the more usual erect posture." Yet postural change is severely restricted in many occupations, especially those that require an individual to sit for several hours in a confined space that prohibits standing or other efforts at changing position. The health of the back is thus put in jeopardy with the consequent reduction in the pumping action that characterizes osmotic disc nutrition.

Nerve Root Entrapment (Sciatica)

Sciatica is usually a direct result of disc herniation. Since 90% of the cases of disc prolapse occur at the level of the lowest two lumbar discs, the referred pain is within the distribution of the sciatic nerve, thus the name sciatica. Reports of the frequency with which disc degeneration leads to sciatica vary tremendously. Some have suggested that about 75% of cases of degenerative disc disease involve foraminal narrowing and that about 40% of cases with foraminal narrowing show signs of nerve root involvement [37]. Others have found nerve root pressure to be much less frequent [38-40]. Although the disc has enjoyed an era of popularity as a specific explanation for referred pain ever since the landmark study by Mixter and Barr in 1934, it is now recognized that a herniation may not be a prerequisite for radicular pain. Root entrapment syndrome may affect the lumbar root in the foraminal canal, while disc prolapse tends to affect the root in the central canal and in its lateral recesses[42]. The nature of pain caused by foraminal compression may be different, tending to be severe, constant and unrelieved by bed rest. The precise distribution of leg pain varies in accordance with the root involved. It usually commences as a dull pain in the back of the thigh or in the buttock, but can later involve the posterior and lateral aspects of the calf, as well as the heel and sole of the foot.

Calliet lists four conditions which contribute to the narrowing of the intervertebral foramina: an approximation of the pedicles due to disc narrowing, osteophyte formation (spurs), osteoarthritis of the facet joints, and thickening of the ligamentum flavum [5]. As a result of these abnormalities, the nerve root is either compressed directly, or tethered and stretched over a protrusion. Postures including standing, walking and reaching overhead can produce pain, as can excessive flexion (most notably seen in a straight-leg raise test) which stretches the nerve and dura over the tissues encroaching upon the foramen.

The anatomy of the nerves make them especially vulnerable to compression. As Mooney points out, the spinal nerve root is different from a peripheral nerve root in that is has no protective epineurium to resist mechanical stress [42]. Instead, it is encased in a flimsy gauze-like pia, allowing maximum diffusion of cerebrospinal fluids, which supply up to 58% of the root's nutrition. Inflammation and scarring (fibrosus) can easily restrict the entrance of nutrients, causing a chemical imbalance possibly resulting in nerve root pain. The reader will be careful to note that this explanation is purely biochemical in nature, having nothing to do with the mechanical aspects of back pain. It indicates the potential for pain to be initiated without structural injury to the disc, ligaments or muscles.

These theories were investigated by Porter et al. in an evaluation of 2360 patients attending a back clinic, from which 249 (10.5% of the entire population) were selected for a group testing positive for root entrapment[41]. Selection was based upon the following criteria: severe and constant root pain, pain unrelieved by bed rest, minimal tension signs, and patients over 40 years of age. The size of this group is contrasted with 9% of the patients having a symptomatic disc lesion, 7% of the patients with neurogenic claudication, and 18% with back and referred pain.

A number of important findings emerge from the report. The high incidence of disc narrowing among the selected group suggest that previous disc pathology is a major cause of this root entrapment syndrome. A previous history of back pain, often many years before, was recorded in 80% of these patients. Porter speculates that "ligamentous changes and soft tissue scarring from previous disc lesion reduced the available space for the nerve root... the degenerative changes of bone and soft tissue so altered the root canal that the nerve root with restricted space or restricted excursion became vulnerable to trauma." Significantly, Porter also concluded that the central canal of patients with root entrapment is nearly the same as the general population. Based upon ultrasound measurements, there is no evidence that this syndrome of nerve root entrapment is related to central canal size, supporting the assertion that the mechanism of pathology need not involve disc herniation or other aspects of spinal stenosis.

Considering the inflammatory component of back pain, Jayson [43] takes the theory even farther with a hypothesis focusing on the deposits of fibrin associated with scar-tissue formation and neural inflammation. According to Jayson, fibrin is normally cleared as chronic inflammation and fibrosus resolve within an acute time period. Yet in some instances, "there is a persistence of fibrin because of a defect in fibrinolytic activity, perhaps secondary to the damage itself or other unknown factors. The failure to clear fibrin leads to persistence of chronic inflammation and fibrosis and chronic back pain." Interestingly, smoking is associated with reduced fibrinolytic activity, which corresponds well to the association of smoking and low back pain discussed earlier in the book.

Spencer et al. investigated the neural elements of back pain in a different manner, based upon a study of the anatomy and fixation of the lumbar nerve roots [44]. He explains "disc protrusion as a necessary but not sufficient condition to produce sciatica symptoms." Sciatic pain will be produced only when a protrusion contacts a nerve root that is relatively immobile, wherein the extrathecal nerve root is stretched taut over the protrusion. In other words, "a contact force may be applied to the extrathecal nerve root by a disc protrusion only if it is relatively fixed anteriorly in the spinal canal (by the dural ligaments)... A disc protrusion will not generate a contact force on an untethered nerve root." This explanation clearly lends support to the widely recognized lack of positive correlation between the magnitude of a disc protrusion and the signs and symptoms of sciatica, indicating why some disc protrusions are totally asymptomatic.

Spencer goes on to develop a convincing hypothesis that explains how pressure can be applied to the nerve root by a protrusion without compression of the nerve against the posterior elements of the lumbar vertebra, implicating the dural ligaments as the primary cause of root tension. Since the dural ligaments are the primary support linkage between the extrathecal nerve root and the vertebral periosteum and longitudnal ligament, it is demonstrated that the dural ligaments may play a dual role in the pathogensis of sciatica. Pain can result from the tethering of the nerve roots over a disc protrusion, affecting not only the local area, but also by transmitting nerve pressure via the tractioning of the posterior longitudnal ligament and vertebral periosteum.

Arachnoiditis

Although most cases of sciatica are attributed to nerve root compression (a biomechanical etiology), radicular pain referred from the low back to the lower extremities can also be caused by neural inflammation. Arachnoiditis is an example of biochemical pathology, and a potent source of back pain. Spinal arachnoiditis has been recognized as a pathologic entity for the past 85 years since the first report by Spiller in 1903 [45]. As the term suggests, the pathology is characterized by inflammation of the arachnoid membrane enveloping the central nervous system. This membrane is a particularly delicate structure which responds to even minimal trauma. Several etiologies have been proposed, including infection, trauma, foreign bodies, and allergic reaction. However, chemical reaction due to some myelographic imaging dyes and trauma from surgical procedures are by far the leading causes of arachnoiditis. The symptoms of this entity are sparce, distinguished by complaints of constant low back pain with or without leg pain and markedly aggravated by activity. While there is a surprising paucity of definitive motor weakness, one frequently observes positive straight-leg raising, tenderness of the sciatic nerves and the sciatic notch, limitation of range-of-motion of the trunk, and paravertebral muscle spasm. Although the clinical presentation of symptoms is relatively clear-cut, definitive medical diagnosis is much more complicated, as diagnosis usually requires either direct surgical observation of the caudal nerve roots or an unequivocal imaging study.

The chronology of arachnoiditis is one of progressive neural atrophy. It begins with inflammation of the pia-arachnoid, characterized by hyperemia and nerve root swelling in the cauda equina. At this stage, the fibrous and elastic material of the arachnoid membrane is just beginning to deposit fibroelastic strands of collagen between the nerve root and their pia-arachnoid coating. As the collagen deposits proliferate, the nerve roots no longer swell but become adherent to their pia-arachnoid sheaths and the sheaths to each other. The last phase is adhesive arachnoiditis, where the pia-arachnoid becomes markedly thickened by excessive collagen deposit. The nerve roots become ischemic and atrophy. Thickening of the sub-arachnoid space can occur at this stage.

Oil-based and ionic water-soluble myelography has been implicated in the development of arachnoiditis. An intervening operation for disc herniation may only worsen the condition. The literature has demonstrated a varying frequency of arachnoiditis following myelography, depending upon the type of contrast media used and/or the number of back surgeries. Benner et al. found the combination of oil-based myelography and spinal surgery as the probable cause of arachnoiditis in 62 of 68 patients diagnosed with the pathology [46]. The authors remark: "The combination of a cellular response, increased protein, residual oil, and the possibility of even minimal transdural operative trauma, would produce a clinical setting similar to those conditions that consistently produce arachnoiditis in experimental models."

Yet oil-based myelography is by no means the only contrast media that causes an inflammatory reaction. In fact, the use of any myelographic dye, whether oil or water soluble can trigger arachnoiditis. Some dyes do appear to be safer than others. Consider these statistics: Methiodal sodium myelography has been linked to an incidence rate of radiographically-confirmed arachnoiditis in 16.5% to 35% of non-operated patients. Positive findings were also found in 8% to 47% of patients receiving meglumine iothalamate, and in 0% to 36% injected with meglumine iocarmate. For those patients operated on between myelographies, the corresponding incidence rate of arachnoiditis ranges from 42% to 75% of those receiving methiodal sodium, 25% to 53% of those receiving meglumine iothalamate, and 42% to 73.5% of patients receiving meglumine iocarmate [47,48]. The track record of iophendylate (also known as Pantopaque) is so disastrous that use of this medium has been restricted in the Scandinavian countries and completely forbidden by law in Sweden. Pantopaque is still used in the United States in certain instances.

Although arachnoiditis occurs frequently and can be radiologically very impressive, most of the patients are asymptomatic. The incidence of symptomatic arachnoiditis where radiological findings are positively correlated to patient's complaints is radically lower than the preceding statistics would indicate. For example, a review by Shaw et al. of 7600 spinal investigations with contrast found the incidence of symptomatic arachnoiditis after myelography to be only 1% [49]. Similar results were documented by Thomalske in a series of 1000 consecutive herniated discs, where an overall incidence rate of 1.5% was noted [50].

The common denominator shared by all of the media noted earlier is the ease with which they are able to diffuse through the sub-arachnoid space. Because of significant osmotic properties, these dyes mix with the cerebral spinal fluid during imaging and ultimately penetrate the arachnoid area, initiating the inflammation process. One contrast media proven to resist diffusion is the non-ionic water soluble metrizamide (Amipaque). In fact, the safety of metrizamide is so widely accepted that is has become the uncontested media of choice for myelographic examination. One need only compare the records of arachnoiditis incidence attributed to contrast media to appreciate why this is true. Hansen et al. analyzed 256 repeat myelograms in 192 patients which could be compared with original myelograms in an effort to evaluate the development of adhesive arachnoiditis attributed to metrizamide and other contrast media[51]. Radiological signs were found in 5 of 46 cases (11%) after methiodal sodium myelography, in 24 of 96 cases (25%) after iothalamate meglumine, in 7 of 12 cases (58%) after iocarmate meglumine, and in 7 of 10 cases (70%) after iodophendylate. None of the 90 metrizamide myelographies showed evidence of adhesive arachnoiditis. It was found that the occurrence of arachnoiditis was dependent on the doses of water soluble contrast media --

the higher the dose, the greater the incidence of adhesive arachnoiditis. Furthermore, a subsequent operation tended to increase the frequency of arachnoiditis, as did increasing time intervals between the original and subsequent myelograms. The safety of metrizamide myelograms is confirmed by Skalpe, who found just one case of arachnoiditis among 77 repeat myelographies [48]. For further information concerning the track record of metrizamide and other contrast media, the reader is referred to the Diagnosis chapter.

Spondylolysis and Spondylolisthesis

One form of vertebral pathology that has fascinated medical researchers for many years is spondylolisthesis, a process characterized by the forward shift of one vertebra on another. The term was coined by Kilian in 1854, derived from the Greek words "spondylos" meaning vertebra, and "olisthesis" meaning a slipping or falling. In its most prevalent form, spondylolisthesis is generally the result of a defect or fracture ("lysis" in Greek) of the pars interarticularis, the narrow bridge of bone between the lumbar superior and inferior articular facets. (Figure 2-1) The pathology was first described in 1782 by Herbinaux, a Belgian obstetrician who noted that there were times when a bony prominence in front of the sacrum caused problems with delivery. Lambi demonstrated the deterioration of the pars in 1855, the most common source of the condition, while Neugebauer in 1881 was the first to demonstrate that slippage can occur by elongation of the pars, without fracture. Spondylolisthesis is reported to have an incidence in the general population of 3% to 5%, with a vertebral slip

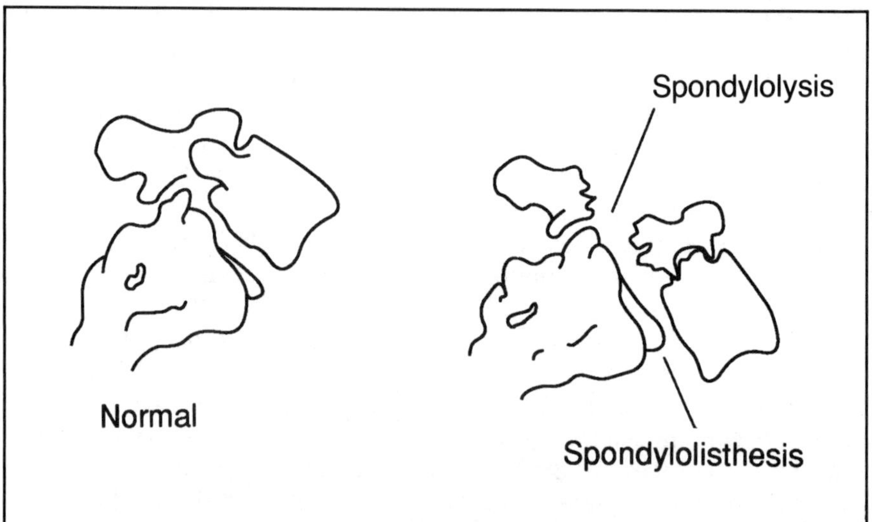

Fig. 2-1: Spondylolysis is a break in the posterior elements of a vertebra. Spondylolisthesis is a slipping forward of one vertebra on another.

usually not greater than 25 to 30 degrees [52-55]. The pathology in adults is associated with decreased mobility of the lumbar spine and a slightly awkward body posture. Contributing to the mystique enshrouding low back etiology, it has been determined that approximately one-half of all patients presenting evidence of the condition are asymptomatic.

The classification of spondylolisthesis includes five primary conditions, derived from previous classifications published by various authors [56,57]. After a brief listing of the various categories, special attention will be given to the three most prevalent types of spondylolisthesis: dysplastic, isthmic and degenerative.

Categories of Spondylolisthesis

I. Dysplastic (congenital). In this type, congenital abnormalities of the upper sacrum or the arch of L5 permit the olisthesis to occur.

II. Isthmic. The lesion is in the pars interarticularis, commonly referred to as spondylolysis by many researchers. Three types can be identified: a. Lytic or fatigue fracture of the pars; b. Elongated but intact pars; c. Acute fracture of the pars.

III. Degenerative. Due to long-standing intersegmental instability.

IV. Post-traumatic. Due to fractures in areas of the bony hook other than the pars.

V. Pathologic. Generalized or localized bone disease.

Dysplastic spondylolisthesis is most likely to produce tight hamstrings. The pars may remain unchanged, elongate or come apart. If it does elongate or fracture, it will be quite difficult to distinguish from Type II A and B. Wynne-Davies et al. have indicated a strong genetic influence, documenting a 33% incidence among relatives with the disorder [58].

Unlike the Dysplastic Type, the basis for Isthmic spondylolisthesis is a defect in the pars, the weakest part of the neural arch. Type A Lytic is a result of stress or fatigue fracture of the pars, and the most common type below the age of 50. The national incidence rate is approximately 5% to 6% in adult Caucasian males, and 2% to 3% in adult Caucasian females. Significantly, it has been demonstrated that a strong hereditary component exists, as one study presented an incidence rate of 15% for the close relatives of patients with isthmic spondylolisthesis [59,60]. Others have observed a 30% incidence among family members. For instance, in a study of 400 school children aged 6, Baker found that 28% of parents presented the same pars defect observed in their children [53]. Other racial differences have been reported, most notably an incidence rate as high as 50% for some Eskimo communities north of the Yukon, possibly attributed to unusual postural stress and a high accident rate [61]. This can be compared to a rate of less than 3% for some black populations [62]. In many individuals with spondylolysis the defect produces no symptoms.

When it does occur, the age group between 5 and 7 appear to be more prone to injury than other groups, possibly due to fatigue fractures from repeated trauma, a consequence of engaging in activity at a time when the intervertebral disc is more elastic and the neural arch may not be completely ossified.

While the true causes of the pathology are unclear, the slippage of the vertebra almost always occurs at the lowest lumbar levels, with 70% of cases occurring at the L5-S1 junction, and 25% at L4-L5. Hence, pain is generally isolated to the low-back, as the normal lumbar lordosis is altered. Under normal conditions, numerous support structures prevent forward sliding on all four sides of the vertebra, as they are stabilized by healthy articular facets and pars, the longitudnal ligaments, annular fibers and normal intradiscal pressure. Considerable force must occur to cause slippage. Three kinds of forces have been implicated in the displacement of the vertebra, as noted by Farfan et al: shearing force, flexion overload and rotational torque [63]. Shearing action is dependent upon the lumbosacral angle (L5-S1), which is generally in the range of 30 to 45 degrees, tilted downward. The natural tendency is for the L5 vertebra to slide downward as the support structures around it weaken. Forward flexion overload causes friction between the superior and inferior facet joints, leading to shearing stress and ultimate fracture and separation of the pars interarticularis. The same outcome is possible with excessive rotational forces.

Such forces are commonly experienced by young athletes, with the literature implicating gymnasts, football players (especially interior linemen) and weight lifters as particularly vulnerable to vertebral displacement due to hyperextension and flexion [64]. For example, a 1979 study by Dominquez found that one-third of all National Football League interior linemen have spondylolisthesis, according to team physicians [65]. It is suggested that as the lineman drives forward from a three-point stance, attempting to push the opponent backward, the lumbar spine is extended in a position which converts more of the force of the collision to shearing energy, leading to injury of the pars articularis. Similarly, the lifting of heavy weights to overhead positions, especially with the trunk in a flexed position, causes very high shear forces to be applied to the lumbar vertebra. A high rate of backache is also seen in gymnastics, which is likely attributed to the hyperlordotic posture seen in many stunts and to the extreme flexibility necessary to perform vaulting, dismounts, flips and other maneuvers. The incidence of spondylolysis in a study of 100 female gymnasts was 11%, as indicated by Jackson [66].

Spondylolisthesis of the degenerative kind is considered by Moe to be the most common pathological condition [56]. There is no pars defect, and the slippage is usually not greater than 30%. What makes the condition uniquely Type III is the advanced degeneration of the facet joints and disc. Moe theorizes that the straight, stable lumbosacral joint puts increased stress on the articular joint between L4 and L5, leading to hypermobility and degeneration of the articular processes and disc. Ultimately, this could result in localized spinal stenosis and possible compression of the cauda equina.

Whether or not spondylolisthesis causes low back pain is a matter of intense debate. Horal, Hult and Torgerson [24,25,67] have each demonstrated an increased incidence of low-back pain when spondylolisthesis was present, while Rowe and Stanton-Hicks [68,69] have observed no such relationship. Nachemson has concluded that spondylolysis with spondylolisthesis is not related to back pain in any greater incidence than in a group of healthy controls. Moe emphasizes that not every patient with this condition suffers from low back pain, claiming to have seen many patients with very severe degrees of spondylolisthesis between 75% to 100% who have been totally asymptomatic.

Osteoarthritis

A degenerative disease of the spinal joint cartilage that affects the facet joints, osteoarthritis has been implicated in the etiology of lumbar pain. Aging causes cartilage loss and the formation of osteophytes, narrowing the joint space between the inferior and superior facets. The gliding action between the two surfaces is consequently disrupted, as the facet surface becomes increasingly abrasive and worn down. The by-product of degeneration is progressively reduced mobility and potentially painful back spasms. Besides degenerative involvement, one must also consider congenital malformation -- most commonly facet tropism. The condition is characterized by asymmetric facet development, thereby disrupting the normal process of load-bearing. The result may be pain, both localized and radicular, and acceleration of the degenerative process in the joint, leading to chronic pain.

It must be noted, however, that these changes are as common in healthy controls as they are in patients with back pain. Flor et al. writes that "such structural changes have been found to be related to age, overweight, scoliosis, and hyperlordosis and may consequently be viewed as a normal aging process and related to strain on the spine. These changes may occur secondary to disc degeneration but cannot be considered as the sole etiological factor for back pain since spinal osteoarthritis is often asymptomatic" [27]. An autopsy report by Levin revealed that 90% of individuals over the age of 45 had osteoarthritis in the lumbar spine and that more joints were affected as age increased [70].

Even so, Lawrence reports that among a sample group suffering from sciatic pain of at least three months duration, 19% of the males were diagnosed with Grade 3-4 arthritis of the lumbar facet joints, compared with 7% of those with Grade 0-1 [4]. The pathology has also been found to occur with greater than expected frequency in miners by Caplan et al. [71] and Kellgren [72]. In a review of the epidemeology of low back pain, Kellsey and White conclude that "degeneration in the intervertebral discs, spondylolisthesis, and lumbosacral transitional vertebrae increase the likelihood of occurence of osteoarthrosis... Age remains the best predictor of osteoarthrosis of the lumbar spine, and mechanical stress is undoubtedly involved as well" [73].

A study by Giles et al. suggests that a miniscule intra-articular synovial protrusion (also known as intravertebral menisci) projecting from the facet joint can be a source of irritation and resultant reflex muscle spasm [74]. The protrusions are described as vascular, fat-filled synovial folds, found at all vertebral levels but best developed in the lumbar region. Although nerve fibers have never been demonstrated within the protrusions, it is known that the facet joint capsule is well innervated, and the author believes it is reasonable to assume the presence of certain nerve fibers. Since the position of the protrusion makes it vulnerable to being nipped between bone and ligament or between the articular cartilages by a sudden twist of the joint, it is also likely to cause low-back pain if the projection becomes entrapped or stretched by the surrounding anatomy. (Figure 2-2)

In support of this theory is a report by Kos et al. who agrees that protrusions are capable of causing "vertebral block" given the scenario described above[75]. Likewise, Lewit confirms that such a protrusion could become impinged upon and imprisoned between the articular surfaces, thereby mechanically interfering with movement, leading to pain and muscle spasm [76]. This etiology has also been accepted by Zukschwerdt [77], Bourdillon [78] and Engel [79] in a number of low-back pain patients.

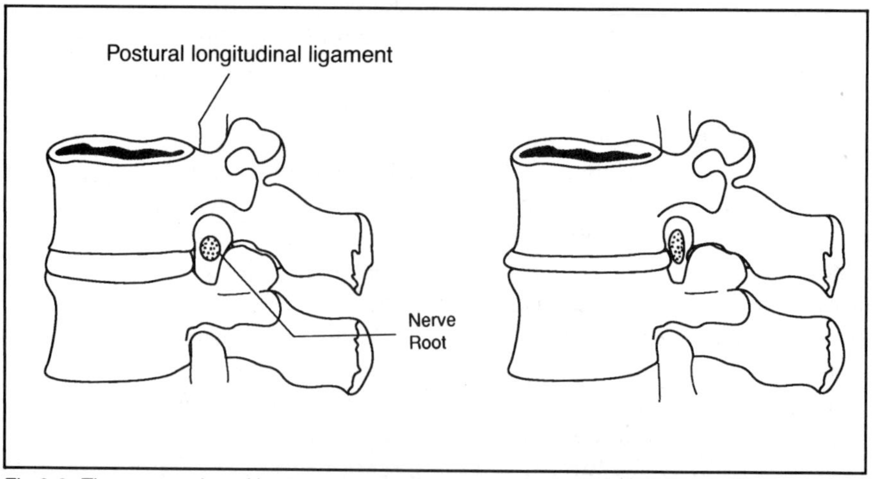

Fig 2-2: The progression of lumbar degenerative change is depicted in the two pictures above. The left figure shows two normal vertebra with a normal disc. The nerve root has adequate room to exit from the foramen. On the right, the disc has settled causing posterior bulging with reduction in size of the foramen and consequent compression of the nerve root.

Lumbar Spinal Stenosis

Stenosis, or narrowing of the vertebral canal, is most commonly observed in the lower lumbar area, attributed to both congenital and degenerative factors. In many cases, the diameter of the spinal canal will often determine which individuals will suffer from back pain. Generally speaking, the literature indicates that those persons with wide canals are more capable of sustaining disc bulging, herniation, hypertrophic ridging into the spinal canal, spondylolisthesis, post-fusion bony extrusion or other degenerative changes that encroach into the neural space, compared to their counterparts with narrow canals that simply lack the space to accommodate the penetration of soft-tissue. Compression of the spinal nerve roots is the end result, often presenting as "psuedo claudication" with pain in one or both legs when walking. Pain may be experienced even when walking a short distance or standing in one position, described by patients as a rubbery feeling in the legs. The condition is also associated with numbness and paraesthesia. Narrowing may be present at birth, as Verbiest reports in his morphological studies [80].

Others argue that certain growth patterns such as hypertrophy of the laminae and articular processes, combined with such degenerative changes as spondylosis, facet impingement, neural arch osteophyte protrusion and disc herniation increase the progression of canal narrowing, even in a congenitally normal vertebral column. Vanharanta comments: "Osteoarthrosis, with its attendant hypertrophy, tends to diminish the space available within the canal and foramina, and this phenomenon is etiologically distinct from the dimensions which are genetically determined[81]." Aiken does acknowledge that significant disc herniation or spondylosis, even in a normal canal, can cause psuedoclaudication. He also states that "It is controversial as to how frequently symptomatic lumbar stenosis actually can be attributed to congenital predisposition [82]".

Of more immediate concern is the relationship between a stenotic lumbar spinal canal and the incidence of low back pain. Considering the degenerative influences of various occupational risk factors, is it possible to isolate a specific worker population that is most vulnerable to stenotic-induced lumbar pain? Macdonald et al. attempted an answer to this question in a study of the relationship between spinal canal diameter and back pain in coal miners [83]. Ultrasound was used to measure the canal diameters of 204 miners between the ages of 50 and 60 years. After a three year follow-up exam, the total number of work days lost due to back pain were compared with the canal measurements. Of the days off work, 32% were lost by the 22 miners with the narrowest spines (below the tenth percentile). The widest canals occurred in those miners having no history of back pain, while the narrowest occurred in those who had retired with a history of back pain.

Macdonald concludes: "The present study suggests that the size of the spinal canal is a factor that contributes to a subject's vulnerability to develop back pain. It supports the observations of Verbeist that many patients requiring spinal surgery have narrow canals [84]. Symptoms associated with a disk lesion also tend to be more disabling if the patient has a narrow canal" [85]. Brown has also reported that in his experience with disc excision, he has almost never encountered a normal spinal canal in those individuals who suffer from back pain [16]. Likewise, Forsberg et al. verified the increased probability of backache with stenosis, based upon the results of surgical treatment of disc herniation [86]. It was found that 12 patients who recovered uneventfully had a significantly broader canal than 10 patients having comparatively narrower canals and still suffering from pain. (Figure 2-3)

Porter concluded that the size of the lumbar canal is a primary component in the generation of both disc pathology and nerve compression, based upon a review of 700 subjects [87]. Ultrasound measurements demonstrated that the majority of patients having disabling disc symptoms had a narrow canal in addition to disc pathology as 56% of 154 patients with disc symptoms were below the tenth percentile for young people. Additionally, 30% of 78 patients diagnosed as having root entrapment had canals below the tenth percentile of the 50 to 65 year old miners, nurses and sedentary workers. It is calculated that a subject whose canal measurement is below the tenth percentile is four times more likely than the rest of the population to have root entrapment

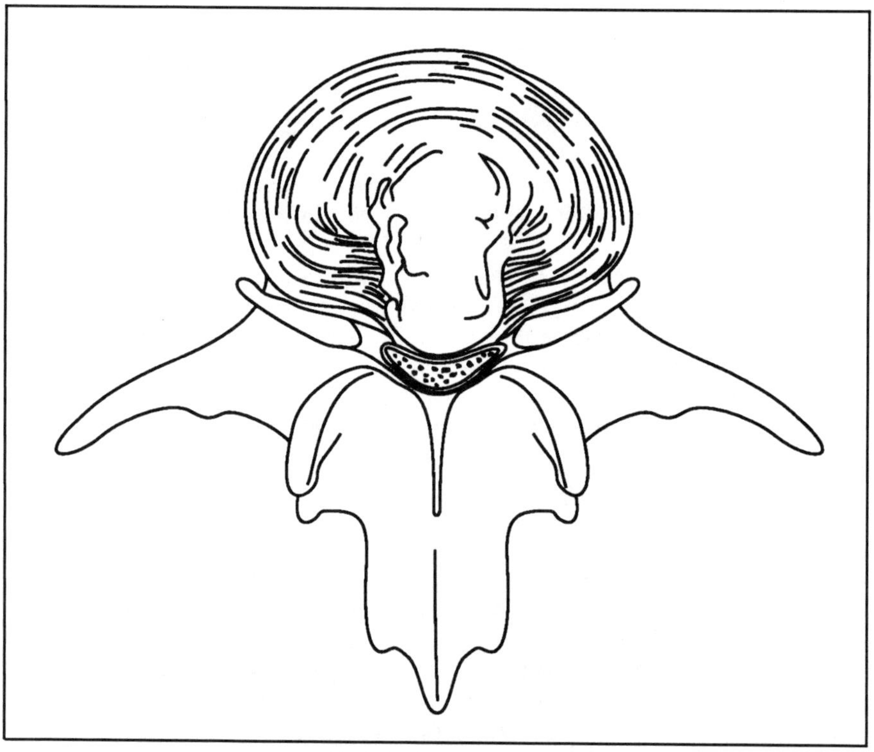

Fig 2-3: Herniated Disc

symptoms, which increases to 11 times in the presence of a disc lesion. Significantly, almost one-half of the 138 patients who had claudication were miners. Furthermore, it was observed that miners working underground for three and four decades had spinal canals slightly wider than men working sedentary jobs. It is speculated this is a result of occupational self-selection, where those miners with troublesome narrow spines have been selected out of the industry in pursuit of other employment.

A similar finding was demonstrated in a study which compared the size and shape of the lumbar vertebral canal with various categories of occupation and work load among 77 men and 118 women having a history of low-back pain [81]. Unlike the coal miner study, the objective of this investigation was to examine the linkage between work activity and narrowness of the canal, based upon the hypothesis that where occupational work load increased the risk of osteoarthritis, narrowing of the intervertebral and interarticular distance would be apparent. The subjects were classified into four groups: white-collar workers, farm workers, industrial workers and service workers. X-ray measurements were taken of the interpedicular and interarticular distance, as well as the anteroposterior foraminal diameter.

Only one of the supposed work-spinal narrowness relationships was proven statistically significant – the degree of physical activity at work. The men who presented a history of heavy manual work had significantly smaller anteroposterior foraminal distances at L5 than their counterparts working in less physically demanding industries. A similar observation was noted in female farm workers, where interarticular distance was shorter than in those working in less strenuous female occupations. No statistical differences in vertebral measurements were found in either men or women whose jobs required paced work, repetitive movements at work, stooped posture, lifting or carrying heavy objects, or vibration. The only exceptions were a statistical significance for men in the stooped posture category (only at L5), and at L3 for the lifting and carrying of heavy objects. Vanharanta explains the mixed results by noting that the subjects did not represent an occupational cross-section of the population, since they were restricted to a sample with significant back pain.

It appears that spinal stenosis is an uncertain factor in the etiology of back pain. In fact, it is probably safe to say that none of the degenerative symptoms discussed – disc degeneration and herniation, spondylolysis, spondylolisthesis, or osteoarthritis – can be definitively considered as the source of pain. Flor and Turk summarize the controversy surrounding the effects of degenerative forces on the spinal system with the following assessment of the current literature: "It remains unclear to what extent degenerative changes may be causes or consequences of low-back pain. There is a lack of direct, conclusive evidence for the role of these degenerative changes of the spine in the etiology of chronic low-back pain. All degenerative processes ... are also present in individuals without any back pain whatsoever. It appears that for chronic low-back pain to develop additional factors must be operative" [27].

Skeletal Abnormalities

Skeletal abnormalities include postural deformities and anatomical anomalies, such as scoliosis and leg-length asymmetry. Each will be evaluated as as potential cause of pain

Scoliosis

Idiopathic scoliosis is the most prevalent form of lateral deviation of the spine, occuring during three stages of childhood growth – infantile, juvenile and adolescent [56]. The etiology is unknown, but has been recognized as a disease for more than a century. Prior to the 1900s, medical research had attributed the etiology of the disease to the postural positioning of the body. More current research has investigated a wide variety of factors possibly influencing the course of spinal deviation, including studies on operative disturbance of bone and spinal ligaments [88], metabolism of connective tissue [89], enzymatic factors, tendon, ligament and joint elasticity, vertebral rotation, and genetic factors [90,91]. Others speculate that the only legitimate etiological explanation is based on inheritance, drawing upon the observation that the disease is found in twins, families, and siblings more frequently than the general population.

Numerous studies have documented the prevalence of scoliosis, almost entirely based upon chest x-rays taken for tuberculosis screening and school health screening. Several findings will be discussed in this section, allowing the reader an opportunity to evaluate the variety of conclusions offered by the literature. It will be demonstrated that the bulk of research indicates a 4% to 5% incidence of scoliosis in North American school children aged 12 to 14, with girls having a significantly greater probability for progressive deformity.

One study evaluated 3064 students at a public school near Seattle, Washington [92]. Composed of an equal number of boys and girls in the seventh, eighth and ninth grades, it was found that 1.6% had confirmed scoliosis. Girls were twice as likely as boys to present positive results (2.1% incidence versus 1.1%). In a review of 50,000 people, Shands et al. noted a scololiosis of 10 degrees or more in 1.9% of those over the age of 14, and a deformity of at least 20 degrees in 0.5% of the sample group [93]. Results of a population of 3299 female students from Australia revealed at least minimal signs of scoliosis in 5.9% of the group [94], while Strayer [95] found a 7% incidence in a review of chest x-rays from 928 women entering a hospital for childbirth. The examination results of both Shands and Strayer used minifilm x-rays in the assessment of scoliosis, an important distinction when one considers the limitations of the procedure: underpenetration of the spine and lack of visualization of the spine.

One of the highest reported incidence rates was reported by Brooks et al. in a screening of 3492 school children from Los Angeles [96,97]. Results indicated a rate of 13.6%, with females having a rate 1.5 times greater than the male population. Furthermore, it was found that the most common abnormal curvature was in the thoracolumbar region. Another study demonstrated one of the very few findings on racial differences and scoliosis. In a review of both white and black students from Johannesburg, South Africa, Segil found curvature in excess of 10 degrees with clinically significant rotation to be prevalent in 2.5% of the white student body, compared with only 0.03% of the African student body [98]. The differences are considered to be highly significant.

A more detailed evaluation of 14,900 students between the ages of 12 to 14 years old from Montreal, Canada was carried out by Drummond et al. [99]. It was determined that 5.5% (821 students) of those screened were believed to present signs of a definite scoliosis. Of the 821 positively diagnosed, 610 had a structural scoliosis of 5 degrees or more with rotational deformity, nearly all of which were considered idiopathic scoliosis. Final results indicated an incidence of spine deformity in 4.6% of the group, and a scoliosis rate of 4.1%. Additionally, the sex incidence was equal in the small curves but was 80% female for curves needing treatment.

Careful consideration of studies like the ones just described have lead many investigators to research the natural history of scoliosis as it relates to progressive curvature. The data has documented evidence that many curves improve spontaneously, but when progression does occur, those with a scoliosis greater than 60 degrees are unlikely to experience correction if the spine is left untreated. According to a two-year review of 146 idiopathic scoliosis by Heine et al, progression always coincided with growth spurts, the degree of progression dependent on the site of the curve [100]. More specifically, the thoracic curves and double curves presented the most progression, while lumbar and thoracolumbar curves had the least amount of deformity. An analysis by Ponsetti et al. [101] followed 335 patients to skeletal maturity, and found that in the absence of any prescribed treatment except exercises, the most severe cases of progression were related to the earliest stages of onset [101]. That is, the earlier the age of onset, the worse the prognosis. James [102] validates the conclusion with his own observation of untreated patients, with the thoracic curves progressing the most and with the worst conditions in those with early onset ages [102]. In a similar review, 560 untreated patients (500 of whom were paralytic, 60 idiopathic) demonstrated an average progression of 75 degrees (15 degrees per year!) from onset of puberty to the end of growth [103]. The average curve was 25 degrees at the onset of puberty (age 10), and the final curve at the end of growth (age 15) was 100 degrees.

In a study of the relationship between scoliosis and consequent back pain, Jackson and Simmons analyzed the incidence of back pain in 197 adults with idiopathic scoliosis in comparison to a control group of 180 adults without spinal deformity [104]. It was determined that the prevalence of back pain was nearly identical for both groups, with 80% of the control group and 79% of the scoliotic group reporting pain. Nachemson supports this finding, reporting no greater incidence in adult scoliotics than in the normal population when adjusted for age and sex [105]. Older studies refute the claim, believing curvature to be associated with pain [106].

The severity of the reported pain was somewhat greater among the scoliotics (51% versus 43%). A questionnaire was distributed to evaluate the long-term clinical course of the back pain. The results indicated a major difference: whereas 53% of the control group had no pain and 11% were better at this time, the scolioisis group did not have a single patient without pain, while 17% were better and 83% were the same or worse.

With an average age of 14 in the scoloisis group, it was observed that the mean age and degree of major curvature increased in an almost linear direction. Additionally, patients with major lumbar curvature had the most pain, while those with major thoracic curvature patterns experienced the least pain. The authors explain this phenomenon, arguing that "as the slow progression of scoliosis occurs.... major complaints localize in concavities of curves where the greatest compressive, shear and torsional forces concentrate. Factors contributing to pain would appear to include facet joint arthritis, degenerative disc disease, spinal stenosis, and nerve root entrapment syndrome, all of which are greatest in the concavity of curves."

Thus far, all of the preceding accounts have dealt exlusively with the incidence of scoliosis among children. Recognizing that much of this book has emphasized the problem of back pain in the industrial worker, it is important to complete the chronology of scoliosis as it affects the adult working population of the industrialized world. Up until this point, nothing has been said about the complications accompanying severe scoliosis, particularly the incidence of cardiorespiratory failure which affects the adult scoliotic.

Nilsonne and Lundgren shed some light on the morbidity of scoliosis in their evaluation of 113 patients who presented signs between the years 1913 to 1918 [107]. The average age at diagnosis was 16, with 88 females and 25 males. A follow-up was done in 1963, finding that of the 102 patients located, 46 had died at an average age of 47. This compares with 9.6 expected deaths for the Swedish population during that time period, an effective mortality rate twice the norm. The cause of death was determined to be pulmonary disease in 60% of the cases, with 16 deaths specifically diagnosed as right heart failure. The outlook for those patients still living at the time of the follow-up was not much better, 90% of them reporting pain and tiredness in in the thoracic or lumbar spine on exertion, and 47% were found to be disabled.

Nachemson also found the mortality rate to be twice that of the general population, based upon his analysis of 130 untreated scoliotic patients seen during 1927-1936 [105]. In a series of 102 idiopathic scoliotics with a follow up of 40 years from maturity, Weinstein and Ponsetti found that 60% of adolescent cases progress more than 5 degrees in adult life, particularly for the group presenting with a thoracolumbar angle between 50 degrees and 75 degrees [108]. Save for one unique case, curves under 30 degrees did not progress significantly. Interestingly, it was also found that right-sided lumbar curves over 30 degrees progressed twice as much as left-sided curves.

Despite the rather dismal scenario just described, the natural history of unfused scoliosis for many is not restricted to increasingly irreversible progression leading to pain. One example is a study of 78 patients followed from skeletal maturity over an average period of 17 years. With special attention to curve deterioration, back pain incidence, and psycholsocial details, Edgar found results which suggest a much more optimistic prognosis than the previous reports [109]. While 44% of the group experienced frequent pain (in contrast to 25% of the normal population), the patients seemed to have achieved successful social adjustment. A large majority of the patients (82%) had married, 96% had some form of employment, and 87% stated that they were satisfied with their work status. A history of depression was found in only 10% of the group. No correlation was found between the site or extent of the pain and the type, balance, rigidity, or progression of the deformity. These findings are much more optimistic than the Swedish studies by Nachemson and Lundgren, and probably diverge from the earlier reports because of the generally poorer health conditions noted during the era of the First World War. Those study groups probably represent a higher incidence of severe infantile deformities, crippling the patient to a more severe degree and leading to greater respiratory complications and morbidity.

In conclusion, consider the following remarks by Moe et al. from his classic text on scoliosis and other back abnormalities: "It has been stated that 'scoliotic adults have no more back pain than the population as whole' and 'arthritic troubles in the adult population are a myth'. We cannot agree with these statements... There can be no question that the adult with a curve of 60 degrees or more stands a great risk for the development of increasing curvature and increasing loss of pulmonary function. It is our opinion that the adult with a throacolumbar curve of 60 degrees or more has a high risk of progression and a high risk of painful arthritic complications" [156].

Leg Length Asymmetry

Unequal leg length is considered a predisposing cause of scoliosis. The generally accepted hypothesis is that short leg length causes a lateral imbalance in erect posture, resulting in pelvic tilt and sacroiliac strain, forcing the spine to compensate by a functional scoliosis. Taillard et al. used EMG measurements to show that an asymmetry of ten millimeters or greater leads to a major increase in the activity of several muscle groups, making it impossible for the patient to maintain a resting standing position [110]. Beal [111,112] concluded that backache is the most common symptom associated with short leg syndrome, while Rush and Steiner [113] determined from x-ray studies that leg length asymmetry was an etiological factor in back problems. Clarke found it to promote the development of chondral damage [114]. Others have implicated short leg of even a few millimeters in the etiology of unilateral hip arthritis [115] and microfracture of the lower extremities [116,117].

The tendency to compensate for asymmetrical leg length by constant lateral bending and axial rotation can result in a functional scoliosis. Such postures are thought to be the most dangerous combination of motion to the disc. Friberg reports that "although the lumbar motion segments are aligned to resist axial torque, the intervertebral joint capsules, as well as any of the numerous musculotendinous ligamentous structures, may suffer from these stresses, resulting in inflammation and pain" [118]. This assessment is backed by Wiltse: "When one considers the asymmetrical stresses that must be imposed on the lowermost discs by short leg, it is difficult to see how it could escape being affected" [119].

Skeletal areas may also be affected by abnormal stress transmitted by the functional scoliosis. For example, Friberg observed a statistically high correlation of back pain and unilateral hip symptoms with leg length inequality [120]. The study was comprised of 653 patients with chronic low-back pain with and without sciatica, 254 patients with chronic unilateral hip pain syndrome, and a control group of 359 healthy Finnish Army men. Leg length measurements were evaluated using the standing roentgenogram method. The results of lumbosacral radiography demonstrated an asymmetry of five millimeters (1/4") or more in 75% of the patients and 44% of the controls. The author notes that the incidence of asymmetry greater than 15 millimeters (3/5") is 5.32 times that of the healthy controls (12% of the low-back group versus 2.2% for controls). As for sciatica, 79% of the 229 patients experienced radicular pain in the longer lower extremity, versus 21% of the pain felt in the shorter lower extremity. The distribution was judged to be highly significant. Those men suffering from chronic hip pain indicated the same pattern – 89% of the cases presented pain on the side of the longer lower extremity, compared with only 11% in the hip of the shorter lower extremity. Again, this was judged to be highly significant. No such lateralizing symptoms were found when leg length inequality was less than five millimeters.

Frymoyer offers the following explanation: "Chronic unilateral low-back and hip symptoms were interpreted to be caused or exacerbated by biomechanical responses, in the lumbar motion segments and hip joints, to the lateral imbalance in the erect posture caused by leg length inequality to the flexible functional scoliosis that subjects the lowermost motion segments to combined torsion and bending loads, and to the various positions of the hip joint of the lower longer extremity." Sciatica is the result of the side bending of the lumbar segments, which causes compression of the concave side of the disc, making the posterolateral side of the disc bulge toward the spinal nerve root on the long leg side.

Many in the medical community believe the case against short leg to be over-rated, pointing to the fact that some degree of asymmetry is present in every human. Indeed, leg length inequality is so common that most variation is considered normal. Moreover, a leg length asymmetry of less than 25 millimeters (1") nearly always escapes observation, and much of the time the subject himself is not aware of the condition. Grundy et al. submitted recent evidence based upon 70 participants which directly contradicts the short leg-back pain linkage [121]. The author concluded that shortening of the lower limb, whatever the anatomical cause, is not a significant causal factor for chronic back pain. Specific reference was made to two individuals having leg length asymmetry in excess of 50 millimeters, neither one of which reported chronic pain.

Muscular Dysfunction

Trigger Points

Muscle spasm and atrophy described in low back pain patients has been viewed as a consequence of the pain, the spinal derangements, or postural faults [27]. Myofascial trigger points are another pathologic factor, located in the skeletal muscle and its associated fascia. Also known as myalgic spots, muscular (non-articular) rheumatism, myogelosis, muscle hardenings and fibrositus, trigger points are self-sustaining and highly irritable [122]. Usually, one event initiates trigger point activity in a muscle and other conditions perpetuate it. Certain structural abnormalities are thought to contribute to myofascial low-back pain.

Muscular Hypertension

By definition, a trigger point is a response to a combination of postural faults, ligamentous strain and other types of tissue inflammation, which will cause an increase in muscle activity[5]. A TP, or chronic muscle spasm, can also be the result of the stress-causality model described by Cohen [123]. The model predicts that increased muscle activity might be based upon tension -- the inability to effectively manage external stress or various levels of pain. As an example, Cohen confirmed that migraine headache patients may be hypersensitive to stimuli and may interpret harmless stimuli as hazardous, possibly leading to spasm in the head and neck musculature during both headache and headache-free periods. The emphasis of this explanation is on the psychological trauma attributed to a chronic condition. How the patient responds to his own pain (whether organic or functional) has a significant influence on muscle relaxation or stress.

A great deal of research has utilized electromyographic (EMG) testing equipment to measure the electrical activity of the paraspinal muscles with the objective of documenting the differential EMG levels between chronic back pain sufferers and healthy control groups. A direct relationship between EMG activity and level of physical task is universally accepted. Of greater interest is the lack of consensus over differences in EMG activity among chronic back cases and healthy controls exposed to identical physical tasks.

Many investigators have published evidence of increased EMG levels caused by organic pathology and/or psychologic stress, presenting significantly higher EMG readings in chronic cases [124-126]. Consistent with the nature of back research, several other notable studies have demonstrated contradictory results. Nachemson investigated the notion of trigger points as it applied to to the paraspinal muscle tissue, observing no pathoanatomical changes which could confirm a relationship between fibrositus (inflammation of the muscle tissue) and low-back pain [127]. Yet the same study, demonstrating a direct relationship between muscle tension and disc pressure, implicated irregularly high muscle tension as a factor leading to disc degeneration, directly contradicting studies which speculated the opposite sequence. Fassbender took a different approach in his analysis of muscular atrophy and degeneration of muscle fiber in hypertensive trapezius muscles [128]. His finding speculated that constant hypertension and subsequent oxygen depletion was the fundamental cause of pathology, possibly leading to constant muscle spasm and upper back pain. Basmajian has presented evidence supporting a negative correlation between a chronic condition and paraspinal muscle activity [129].

Of particular interest is a dissenting opinion by Collins et al., who used a comparative analysis of surface electrode paraspinal EMG activity during different levels of physical tasks and physiological stress to test the theories discussed above [130]. Two groups of eleven volunteer men and women between the ages of 20 and 60 participated. The chronic low back group required that each subject have a minimum six month history of seeking medical treatment, while the controls were accepted only if they had no previous history of treatment for low-back pain and had not experienced pain during the 12 months prior to participation. The experiment measured EMG during rest, mild, moderate and relatively physically demanding movements, in addition to two psychologically stressful tasks.

Remarkably, the results indicated that the chronic cases had similar or significantly less paraspinal activity than the control group during tasks specifically designed to activate the back muscles. Additionally, an evaluation was completed to test the theories relating chronic back pain to asymmetry in muscle tension level (see Scoliosis section). No group differences were found. Concerning a test of the ability of the participants to perform postures, the only statistically significant difference was maximum bend posture, with more people in the control group able to perform. Finally, it was determined that at no time did the chronic group have a significantly higher tension level than the control group.

If one accepts the finding to be representative of the larger population, then the validity of the irregular EMG-back pain model emphasizing increased muscle activity in the etiology of chronic back pain is called into question. A different mechanism beneath this supposed relationship must be at work. The authors conclude by proposing an alternative explanation in the sequences leading to chronic back pain: "Perhaps a minor injury to the back occurs and the person perceives some limitation and pain in back movement. Increased anxiety over this relatively minor problem leads to improper performance of trunk and pelvic movements. A viscious circle of maladaptive behavioral patterns is produced which results in a hesitancy to perform common movements correctly, which in turn, produces increased pain and more anxiety. Eventually, this inability to properly control the back results in reduced paraspinal muscle activity."

What is one to make of so many conflicting reports? In a review of the current literature dealing with etiology, Flor et al. writes that the "studies that examined the muscle tension levels of back pain patients are equivocal [as] conclusions from these studies are hampered by methodological problems. The current research has failed to demonstrate an unequivocal relationship among muscle spasm, hypertension and pain" [126]. The authors also include an interpretation by Wood and Badley which insightfully summarizes the wide array of confusing theories, contradictory observations and ambiguous conclusions which mark the research of back pain etiology [131].

"We can find little to refute the suspicion that most published work has sought only for evidence consistent with the author's preconceived notions [as] striking inconsistencies tend to be ignored, neglecting the fact that differential morbidity rates between occupational groups can present useful opportunities for a falsification of hypotheses."

Finally, consider this assessment: "If one tries to delineate the possible causes of back pain one must resort to speculation with little empirical basis .... Neither degenerative, nor structural or muscular, nor occupational factors seem to have any clearcut relationship to low back pain. They may contribute to back pain but they to do not seem to be sufficient causes for most chronic back pain. It is probably wrong to look for a single cause of pain. Chronic low back pain should more appropriately be viewed as multiply determined with specific factors achieving etiological significance only by their interaction" [27].

References

1. Mixter WJ, Barr JS: Rupture of the intervertebral disc with involvement of the spinal canal. N Engl J Med 21:210, 1934.
2. Nachemson A: A critical look at the treatment for low back pain. Scan J Rehab Med 11:143-149, 1979.
3. Dillane JB, Fry J, Kalton G: Acute back syndrome – A study from general practice. Br Med J 2:82-84, 1966.
4. Lawrence JS: The epidemiology of low back pain. Current Orthop 1:361-365, 1987.
5. Calliet R: Low Back Pain Syndrome. FA Davis, Philadelphia, 1980.
6. Benn RT, Wood PHN: Pain in the back – An attempt to estimate the size of the problem. Rheumatol Rehab 14:121-128, 1975.
7. Klein AC, Sobel D: Backache Relief: The Ultimate 2nd opinion from backpain sufferers nationwide. Times Books, NY 1985.
8. Steinmann M: The American Medical Association Book of Back Care. Random House, 1982.
9. Rowe ML: Are routine spine films on workers in industry cost- or risk-benefit effective? J Occup Med 24(1):41, 1982.
10. Puschel J: Wassergehalt normalen und degeneraten zwischen Wirbelscheiben. Beitr. Pathol. 84:123-130, 1930.
11. Schmorl G, Junghanns H: Die gesunde und kranke Wirbelseule im Roentgenbild. Thieme, Leipzig, 1932.
12. Fahrni WH: Conservative treatment of lumbar disc degeneration: our primary responsibility. Orthop Clin N Amer 6:93-103, 1975.
13. Lewinnek GE: Management of low back pain and sciatica. Int Anesthesiol Clin 21:61-78, 1983.
14. Twomey LT, Taylor JR: Age changes in lumbar vertebrae and intervertebral discs. Clin Orthop 224:97-104, 1987.
15. Saraste H: Symptoms in relation to the level of spondylolysis. Intern Orthop 10:183-185, 1986.
16. Brown M: The pathology of lumbar disc disease. From Rothmann RH, Simeone FA: The Spine. WB Saunders, 1982, pp. 510-521.
17. O'Connell JEA: Protrusions of the lumbar intervertebral discs. J of Bone and Joint Surgery 38B:8-30, 1951.
18. Weber H: Lubar disc herniations: A prospective study of prognostic factors including a controlled trial. J Oslo City Hosp 28:33-64, 89-120, 1978.
19. Adams MA, Hutton WC: Gradual disc prolapse. Spine 10:524-532, 1985.
20. Nachemson A: Recent advances in the treatment of low back pain. Int Orthop 9:1-10, 1985.
21. Vanharanta H, Sachs V, Spive M: Disc degeneration and leaking of annulus and reproduction of back pain during discography, ACT discographic study. Abstracts of the International Society for the Study of the Lumbar Spine, Dallas, June 1, 1986.

22. Hirsch C, Ingelmark B, Miller M: The anatomical basis for low back pain. Acta Orthop Scand 33:1, 1963.
23. Sachs B, Spive M, Vanharanta H et al: Dallas discogram description: A new classification of CT/Discography. Spine 12:287-294, 1987.
24. Horal J: The clinical appearance of low back disorders in the city of Gothenburg, Sweden. Acta Orthop Scand (Suppl) 118:8-73, 1969.
25. Hult L: Cervical, dorsal, and lumbar spinal syndromes. A field investigation of a non-selected material of 1200 workers in different occupations with special reference to disc degeneration and so-called muscular rheumatism. Acta Orthop Scand 17 (Suppl):1-102, 1954.
26. Hussar AE, Guller EJ: Correlation of pain and the roentgenographic findings of spondylosis of the cervical and lumbar spine. Amer J Med Sci 232:518-527, 1956.
27. Flor H, Turk DC: Etiological theories and treatments for chronic back pain. I. Somatic models and interventions. Pain 19:105-121, 1984.
28. Nachemson A: Pathomechanics and treatment of low back pain and sciatica. In: M. Stanton-Hicks and R. Boas (Eds.), Chronic Low Back Pain, Raven Press, New York, 1982. Pgs 59-70.
29. Sandoval J: Dynamic loading as a possible source of low back disorders. Spine 8:652-658, 1983.
30. Nachemson A, Lewin T, Maroudas A, Freeman MAR: In vitro diffusion of dye through the end-plates and the annulus fibrosus of human lumbar intervertebral discs. Acta Orthop Scand 41:589-607, 1970.
31. Rolander SD, Blair WE: Deformation and fracture of the lumbar vertebral end-plate. Orthop Clin North Am 6(1):75-81, 1975.
32. Brown T, Hansen RJ, Yorra AJ: Some mechanical tests on the lumbosacral spine with particular reference to the intervertebral disc. J Bone Joint Surg 39A:1135-1164, 1957.
33. Freeman MAR: The pathogenesis of primary osteoarthrosis: An hypothesis. In Modern Trends in Orthopaedics Vol 6. Edited by AG Apley. Butterworth, 1972.
34. Frymoyer JW, Pope MH: The role of trauma in low back pain: A review. J Trauma 18(9):628-634, 1978.
35. Hansson T, Roos B: Intraspongious disc herniation and bone mineral content in lumbar vertebrae. 6th Annual meeting ISSLS, Goteborg, May/June 1979.
36. Adams MA, Hutton WC: The effect of posture on diffusion into lumbar intervertebral discs. J Anat 147:121-134, 1986.
37. Lawrence JS: Disc degeneration, its frequency and relationship to symptoms. Ann Rheum Dis 28:121-137, 1969.
38. Palles C, Jones AM, Spillane JD: Cervical spondylosis, incidence and implications. Brain 77:274-289, 1954.

39. Hussar AE, Guller EJ: Correlation of pain and the roetgenographic findings of spondylosis of the cervical and lumbar spine. Am J Med Sci 232:518-527, 1956.
40. Lawrence JS, DeGraaff R, Laine VAJ: Degenerative joint disease in random samples and occupational groups. The Epidemiology of Chronic Rheumatism. Vol I. Edited by JH Kellgren. Oxford, Blackwell, 1963, pgs 98-119.
41. Porter RW, Hibbert C, Evans C: The natural history of root entrapment syndrome. Spine 9:418-21, 1984.
42. Mooney V: Where is the pain coming from? Presidential Address International Society for the Study of the Lumbar Spine. Dallas, 1986. Spine 8:754-759, 1987.
43. Jayson MIV: The inflammatory component of mechanical back problems. Brit J of Rheum 25:210-213, 1986.
44. Spencer D, Irwin GS, Miller JAA: Anatomy and significance of fixation of the lumbosacral nerve roots in sciatica. Spine 8:672-679, 1983.
45. Spiller WG, Musser JH, Martin E: Arachnoidal cysts. Univ Penn Med Bull 16:27-30, 1903.
46. Benner B, Ehni G: Spinal arachnoiditis. The postoperative variety in particular. Spine 3(1):40-44, 1978.
47. Irstam L, Sundstrom R, Sigstedt B: Lumbar myelography and adhesive arachnoiditis. Acta Radiol (Diagn). 15:356-368, 1974.
48. Skalpe IO: Adhesive arachnoiditis following lumbar radiculography with water-soluble contrast agents. Radiology 121:647-651, 1976.
49. Shaw MDM, Russell JA, Grossart KW: The changing pattern of spinal arachnoiditis. J Neurol Neurosurg Psych 41:97-107, 1978.
50. Thomalske G, Galow W, Ploke G: Critical comments on a comparison of two series (100 patients each) of lumbar disc surgery. Adv of Neurosurg 4:22-27, 1977.
51. Hansen EB, Fahrenkrug M, Praestholm J: Late meningeal effects of myelographic contrast media with special reference to metrizamide. Br J of Radiol 51:321-327, 1978.
52. Bailey W: Observations on the etiology and frequency of spondylolisthesis and its precursors. Radiology 48:107-113, 1947.
53. Baker DR, McHollick W: Spondyloshesis and spondylolisthesis in children. Proceedings of the American Academy of Orthopedic Surgeons, 1956. J Bone Joint Surg 38A:933-934, 1956.
54. Roche MB, Rowe GG: The incidence of separate neural arch and coincident bone variations. A summary. J Bone Joint Surg 34A:491- 494, 1952.
55. Rowe ML: Low back disability in industry: Updated position. J Occup Med 13:476-478, 1971.
56. Moe JH, Winter RB, Bradford DS, Lonstein JE: Scoliosis and other spinal deformities. WB Saunders, Philadelphia, 1978.

57. Finneson BE: Low back pain. JB Lipincott, Philadelphia, 1980.
58. Wynne-Davies R, Scott JHS: Inheritance and spondylolisthesis: A radiographic family survey. J Bone Joint Surg 61B:301-305, 1979.
59. Wiltse LL: Spondylolisthesis and its treatment. From Finneson BE: Low back pain. JB Lipincott, Philadelphia, 1980.
60. Yano T, Meyagi S, Ikari T: Studies of familial incidence of spondylolisthesis. Singapore Med J 8(3):203, 1967.
61. Stewart TD: The age incidence of neural arch defects in Alaskan natives, considered from the standpoint of etiology. J Bone Joint Surg 35A:937, 1953.
62. Roche MB, Rowe GG: The incidence of separate neural arch and coincident bone variations. Anat Rec 109:233, 1951.
63. Farfan HF, Osteria V, Lamy C: The mechanical etiology of spodylolsis and spondylolisthesis. Clin Orthop 117:40-55, 1976.
64. Alexander MJL: Biomechanical aspects of lumbar spine injuries in athletes: A review. Canadian J of Appl Sport Sciences 10:1-20, 1985.
65. Dominquez RH: The Complete Book of Sports Medicine. New York, Chalrles Scribner's, 1979.
66. Jackson DW, Wiltse L, Cirincione R: Spondylolysis in the female gymnast. Clin Orthop and Rel Res 117:68-73, 1976.
67. Torgerson WR, Dotter WE: Comparative roentgenographic study of the asymptomatic and symptomatic lumbar spine. J Bone Joint Surg 58A:850-853, 1976.
68. Rowe ML: Disc surgery and chronic low back pain. J Occup Med 7:196-202, 1965.
69. Stanton-Hicks M, Boas R: Chronic Low Back Pain. Raven Press, New York, 1982.
70. Levin T: Osteoarthritis in lumbar synovial joints, a morphologic study. Acta Orthop Scand (Suppl) 73, 1964.
71. Caplan PS, Freedman LMJ, Connelly TP: Degenerative joint disease of the lumbar spine in coal miners — a clinical and x-ray study. Arthritis Rheum 9:693-702, 1966.
72. Kellgren JH: Osteoarthrosis in patients and populations. Br Med J 2:1-6, 1961.
73. Kellsey JL, White AA: Epidemiology and impact of low back pain. Spine 5:133-142, 1980.
74. Giles LGF, Taylor JR: Intra-articular synovial protrusions in the lower lumbar apophyseal joints. Periodical unknown.
75. Kos J, Wolf J: Les menisques intervertebraux et leur role possible dane les blocages vertebraux. Ann Med Physique 15:203-217, 1972.
76. Lewit K: Beitrag zur reversiblen gelenksblockierung. Zeitschr Orthop 105:150, 1968.

77. Zukschwerd L, Emminger E, Beidermann F, Zettel H: Wirbelgelenk und Bandsheibe. Hipokrates, Verlag, Stuttgart, 1955.
78. Bourdillon JF: Spinal Manipulation, (2nd ed) London, William Heinemann Medical Books, Ltd. 1973.
79. Engel RM, Bogduk N: The menisci of the lumbar zygapophyseal joints. In Proceedings of the Anatomical Society of Australia and New Zealand, 18th Annual Conference, May 1980. J Anat 132:296, 1981.
80. Verbeist H: Pathomorphologic aspects of developmental lumbar stenosis. Orthop Clin N Amer 6:177-196, 1975.
81. Vanharanta H, Heliovaara M, Korpi J, Troup JDG: Occupation, work load and the size and shape of lumbar vertebral canals. Scand J Work Environ Health 13:146-149, 1987.
82. Aiken BM, Cohen BS: The role of congenital anomalies in low back pain. MD State Med J, January:38-41, 1983.
83. MacDonald EB, Porter R, Hibbert C, Hart J: The relationship between spinal canal diameter and back pain in coal miners. J of Occup Med 26:23-28, 1984.
84. Verbeist H: Treatment of idiopathic developmental stenosis of the lumbar vertebral canal. J Bone Joint Surg 59B:485-487, 1978.
85. Porter RW, Hibbert C, Wellman P: Backache and the lumbar spinal canal. Spine 5:99-105, 1980.
86. Forsberg L, Walloe A: Ultrasound in sciatica. Acta Orthop Scand 53:393-395, 1982.
87. Porter RW, Hibbert C, Wellman P: Backache and the lumbar spinal canal. Spine 5:99-105, 1980.
88. Langenskiold A, Michelsson JE: The pathogenesis of experimental progressive scoliosis. Acta Orthop Scand, Suppl 59:26, 1962.
89. Langenskiold A, Michelsson JE: Experimental progressive scoliosis in rabbits. J Bone Joint Surg 43B:116, 1961.
90. MacEwen DG, Cowell HR: Familial incidence of idiopathic scoliosis and its implication in patient treatment. J Bone Joint Surg 52A:405, 1970.
91. Winter RB: Scoliosis and growth. From Zorab PA (ed.): Third Symposium Held at the Institute of Diseases of the Chest, Brompton Hospital, London, Nov. 13, 1970. Churchill Livingstone, London, 1971.
92. Walker DG: An evaluation of an external splint for idiopathic structural scoliosis in infancy. J Bone Joint Surg 47B:524-525, 1965.
93. Shands AR, Jr., Eisberg HB: The incidence of scoliosis in the state of Delaware. A study of 50,000 minifilms of the chest made during a survey for tuberculosis. J Bone Joint Surg 37A:1243, 1955.
94. Golomb M, Taylor TKF: Screening adolescent school children for scoliosis. Med J Aust, June 14, 1975, pp. 761-762.

95. Strayer L: The incidence of scoliosis in the post partum female on Cape Cod. Paper presented at the SRS, Wilmington, 1972.
96. Brooks HL, Azen SP, Gerberg E, Brooks R, Chan L: Scoliosis - a prospective epidemiologic study. J Bone Joint Surg 57A:968-972, 1975.
97. Brooks HL, Gerberg E, Mazur H, Brooks R, Nickel RV: The epidemiology of scoliosis - a prospective study. Orthop Rev 1:17-23, 1972.
98. Segil CM: The incidence of idiopathic scoliosis in the Bantu and white population groups in Johannesburg. J Bone Joint Surg 56B:393, 1974.
99. Drummond D, Rogala E, Gurr J: School screening , a community project. Paper presented at the Quebec Scoliosis Society Meeting, Montreal, June, 1976.
100. Heine J, Reher H: Die Progredienz der unbehandelten idiopathischen Skoliose bis Wachstumsabschluss. Z Orthop 113:87-96, 1975.
101. Ponsetti IV, Friedman B: Prognosis in idiopathic scoliosis. J Bone Joint Surg 32A:381-395, 1950.
102. James JIP: Idiopathic scoliosis: The prognosis, diagnosis, and operative indications related to curve patterns and the age of onset. J Bone Joint Surg 36B:36-49, 1954.
103. Duval-Beaupere G: Pathogenic relationship between scoliosis and growth. In Zorab PA (ed.): Proceedings of 3rd Symposium held at the Institute of Diseases of the Chest, London, 1971.
104. Jackson RP, Simmons EH, Stripinis D: Incidence and severity of back pain in adult idiopathic scoliosis. Spine 8:749-756, 1983.
105. Nachemson A: A long term followup study of non-treated scoliosis. Acta Orthop Scand 39:466-476, 1968.
106. Bergofsky EH, Turino GM, Fishman AP: Cardiorespiratory failure in kyphoscoliosis. Medicine 38:263-317, 1959.
107. Nilsonne U, Lundgren KD: Long-term prognosis in idiopathic scoliosis. Acta Orthop Scand 39:466-476, 1968.
108. Weinstein SL, Ponsetti IV: Curve progression in idiopathic scoliosis. J Bone Joint Surg 65A:447-455, 1983.
109. Edgar MA: The natural history of unfused scoliosis. Orthop 10:931-939, 1987.
110. Taillard W, Morscher E: Die Beinlangeunterschiede. Basel, S Karger, 1965.
111. Beal MC: A review of the short-leg problem. JAOA 50(2):109-121, 1951.
112. Beal MC: The short-leg problem. JAOA 76:745-751, 1977.
113. Rush WA, Steiner A: A study of lower extremity length inequality. Am J Roentgenol 55:616-623, 1946.
114. Clarke GR: Unequal leg length -- An accurate method of detection and some clinical results. Rheum Phys Med 11:385-390, 1972.
115. Gofton GP: Studies in osteoarthrosis of hip and leg length disparity. Can Med Assoc J 104:791-799,1971.

116. Friberg O: Leg length discrepancy in stress fractures. J Sports Med Phys Fitness, 1982.
117. Friberg O, Kvist M: Leg length inequality in athletes. (Abstract) Preseneted at the XXII World Congress of Sports Medicine, Vienna 1982.
118. Friberg O: Clinical symptoms and biomechanics of lumbar spine and hip joint in leg length inequality. Spine 8:643-651, 1983.
119. Wiltse LL: The effect of the common anomalies of the lumbar spine upon disc degeneration and low back pain. Orthop Clin N Am 2:569-581, 1971.
120. Friberg, Ora: Clinical Symptoms and Biomechanics of Lumbar Spine and Hip Joint in Leg Length Inequality: Spine, Vol. 8(6) pp 643-651, 1983
121. Grundy PF, Roberts CJ: Does unequal leg length cause back pain. A case controlled study. Lancet 2:256-258, 1984.
122. Myofascial origins of low back pain. I. Principles of diagnosis and treatment. Postgrad Med 73:68-77, 1983.
123. Cohen MJ: Psychophysiological studies of headache: Is there similarity between migraine and muscle contraction headaches? Headache 18:4, 1978.
124. Floyd, WF, Silver PHS: The function of the erectores spinae muscles in certain movements and postures in man. J Physiol 129:184, 1955.
125. Kraus H: Bachache -- Stress and Tension. Simon and Schuster, New York, 1965.
126. Rose DL: The decompensated back. Arch Phys Med 56:51,1975.
127. Nachemson A: Pathomechanics and treatment of low back pain and sciatica. From Stanton-Hicks M, Boas R (eds.): Chronic Low Back Pain, Raven Press, New York, 1982.
128. Fassenbender HG: Pathologie und pathogenese des weichteilrheumatismus. In: A. Weintraub, R Battegay, D Beck, G Kaganas, F Labhardt und W. Mueller (Eds). Psychosomatische Schmerzsyndrome des Bewegungsapparates, Schwabe, Basel, 1975. pgs 137-169.
129. Basmajian JV: Cyclobenzaprine hydrochloride effect on skeletal muscle spasm in the lumbar region and neck: Two double-blind controlled clinical and laboratory studies. Arch Phys Med 59:58, 1978.
130. Collins GA, Cohen MJ, Naliboff BD, Schandler SL: Comparative analysis of paraspinal and frontalis EMG, heart rate, and skin conductance in chronic low back pain patients and normals to various postures and stresses. Scand J Rehab Med 14:39-46, 1982.
131. Wood PHN, McLeish CL: Statistical appendix -- digest of data on the rheumatic diseases. 5. Morbidity in industry, and rheumatism in general practice. Ann Rheum. Dis., 33:93-105, 1974.

CHAPTER 3

The Diagnosis of Low Back Pain

Introduction

Accurate diagnosis is a most important factor in the successful management of low back injuries, especially those cases requiring surgical treatment. An appropriate diagnostic strategy recognizes the importance of the clinical and social setting of the injury, as well as the psychological condition of the patient. Resources spent in assuring an accurate and complete diagnosis are crucial in achieving a successful outcome.

Some authors suggest that diagnostic modalities, such as discography and myelography, be used only if the course of management has already been decided. These authors argue that testing using magnetic resonance imaging (MRI), computed tomography (CT), myelography and discography should not be used to decide if a patient requires surgical intervention. As McCall et al. describes it, "the radiological investigation decides where, not whether, the patient is to be operated" [1]. While each radiographic technique has its place in the evaluation of back injury, it requires skillful clinical judgement to select procedures on the basis of their performance characteristics so that the correct diagnosis is obtained for the least cost.

During the following discussion of the most common diagnostic tools currently utilized, the reader should keep in mind that some studies rely entirely on radiological interpretations in determining the accuracy of CT, myelography or other imaging techniques. A clear distinction is made between such a study and one that utilizes the results of operatively proven pathology in the assessment of the predictability of a given diagnostic modality. When possible, we will discuss in what manner the results of a given study were confirmed.

Imaging Techniques

Roentgenograms (X-rays, Plain Films)

With so many different diagnostic procedures to choose from in today's brave new world of nuclear magnetic resonance imaging and metrizamide-enhanced computed tomography, it is vital that the clinician structure a diagnostic program that begins with standard x-rays, employing high-technology imaging tools only when a treatment strategy has been formulated. The objective of plain films is not to establish the presence of back pain, but to specifically identify the most serious pathologies, such as spondylolisthesis, malignancy and ankylosing spondylitis. Generally speaking, x-rays will reveal the bony and structural abnormalities associated with back pain. Other diseases such as spondylosis, disc degeneration, and nerve root entrapment may cause pain the severity of which bears little relationship to the extent of changes demonstrated on plain films. Exact delineation requires further evaluation, usually by CT or MRI.

Although x-rays have limited use in the imaging of non-mechanical or idiopathic back pain, they can have great value in the management of patients with confirmed lumbar disc disease and can be especially helpful should surgical intervention be required. Plain films allow the physician to establish whether or not lumbar spinal instability is present, and identify other etiological factors potentially related to symptoms. Lastly, they enable the identification of segmentation anomalies, present in up to 30% of all patients, avoiding surgery at the wrong level. Thomas notes that any one of these three conditions, if undetected, could lead to failed disc surgery [2].

The most widely used projections in the screening of the lumbar spine are the standard anteroposterior, lateral, and oblique views, which allow assessment of lumbar alignment, vertebral body size comparison, bone density and architecture, as well as gross evaluation of soft tissue structures [3]. The lateral projection views of the lumbar column are best performed with the patient in the standing or upright position. Such a position provides better visibility of the disc space, as well as spondylolisthesis and scoliosis. Oblique views (45 degrees) of the lumbar spine are used in the detection of unilateral or bilateral spondylolysis. While some claim that this perspective accurately depicts spondylolyis, other studies found oblique x-rays to be useful in only 2.4% of all cases [4]. Thomas recommends that oblique views be eliminated from routine x-ray examination and "reserved for adolescents or young adults with symptomatic spondylolysis or possible acute fracture of the pars interarticularis" [2].

Diseases such as ankylosing spondylitis, spondylolisthesis, spondylolysis with marked defect of the pars interarticularis, narrowing of the disc, facet trophism, fractures, and scoliosis are all readily apparent with plain radiography. Unfortunately, x-rays are unable to obtain adequate detail of the posterior neural arch, an intersection of several pain-producing tissues. Additionally, the difficulty in imaging soft tissue surrounding and within the spinal canal is a significant drawback. The lack of visual clarity is directly responsible for a 31% false-negative rate, far more than the documented levels of CT, myelography and MRI. Surprisingly, x-rays were found to have only a 9% false-positive rate [5]. Yet another limitation is the radiation exposure involved with the procedure. One researcher has calculated that a three-view lumbosacral spine examination produces the same amount of radiation to the ovaries as would a chest radiograph performed daily for up to 98 years [1].

Degenerative changes found on plain films occur equally in non-symptomatic as well as symptomatic individuals. In a roentgenographic comparison of 100 patients with backache and an equal number of healthy controls, Splithoff found that with respect to certain types of lumbar pathology, the control group exhibited a higher incidence rate than those suffering backache[6]. For instance, 3% of normal persons presented signs of spondylolisthesis, compared with 2% of the back pain group. Spinal bifida occulta was found in 6% of normal subjects and 4% of patients with backache. Osteoarthritis was present in 22% of normal patients and 26% of those with backache.

These statistics can be contrasted with the reported abnormalities in 21% of 450 non-symptomatic job applicants, and a rate of 17% in 1000 preemployment examinations for General Motors [7]. A similar distribution is observed by Witt et al, in a study of 238 patients with low back pain and sciatica [8]. Compared to a control group of 66 patients without back pain, no differences in the incidence of spondylosis and disc degeneration were revealed between the two groups. Bailey found that while 5% of a back pain group presented radiographic evidence of isthmic spondylolisthesis, only 0.5% of those with defects complained of low back pain[9]. Additionally, a review of 100 healthy soldiers by Friedman et al. reported that only 20% of the group had normal x-rays of the lumbar spine [10]. Since the literature has indicated that routine x-ray examination is rarely unequivocal, the reader should not be surprised to discover that in a review of 68,000 roentgenograms observed over a ten year period, Nachemson concluded that clinically unsuspected positive findings in patients 20 to 50 years of age were obtained only once in every 2,500 examinations [11].

In a different approach regarding the diagnostic value of x-rays, Frymoyer et al. emphasized the tremendous variability of radiographic interpretation among a group of radiologists and chiropractors given a series of x-rays to evaluate [12]. Ninety-nine subjects were randomly selected for anteroposterior and lateral lumbar radiography, the results of which were independently reviewed by three chiropractors. Only a few observations made by chiropractors could be compared to observations by a radiologist. Interobserver reliability measurements showed that only 6 of 56 variables analyzed produced a high concurrence rate: short leg discrepancy, sacral base angle, Ferguson's weight bearing line, lumbarization, spondylolysis, and spondylolisthesis.

Variables with the lowest levels of reliability were innominate subluxation, shortened pedicles, narrow spinal canal, wedged vertebrae and pelvic rotation. Using a coefficient rating system where the minimum level of reliability had a value of .6 or .7, the greatest coefficient for any of the 56 remaining variables was 0.335, well below the level required to have practical usefulness.

Frymoyer saw no alternative in concluding that "spinal radiographs, whether analyzed by measurements, by a radiologist, or by chiropractors, have minimal value in determining the presence or absence of low-back complaints and, in particular, have no value in epidemiologic studies." We would take issue with Frymoyer and others by noting that ruling out infections, fractures, malignancies, or rheumatic disease is very valuable to a low back pain sufferer. What the above data suggest is that repeated, frequent back x-rays in the absence of significant change in symptoms are not helpful.

Myelography

Myelography was first developed with the introduction of the imaging agent iophendylate (Pantopaque) in 1944, an oil-based contrast dye that allows a more exact localization of disc herniation and spinal nerve compromise. While the high iodine content of Pantopaque renders it easily visible even in the thickest anatomical parts of the back, the mixture of iophendylate and spinal fluid with blood, steroids, or even air may incite development of arachnoiditis. Arachnoiditis is probably the most troublesome complication of myelography. It is a crippling disease with no cure, often characterized by transient violent spasms in the legs, muscle cramps, and increased radicular pain. Additionally, the high viscosity of this oil-based contrast requires the use of large gauge needles for injection and removal of material, often the cause of postspinal puncture headache.

Various water-soluble agents have been tried in an attempt to limit some of the dangerous side-effects which commonly accompany the injection of contrast material into the spinal canal. In 1968, the nonionic water-soluble contrast medium, metrizamide (Amipaque) was developed in Norway in an attempt to limit the myelographic complications associated with Pantopaque. After rigorous testing, the FDA approved the agent for general use in the United States. Despite minor toxicity, (including frequent occurrance of headaches, nausea, and vomiting after injection) metrizamide has all but replaced Pantopaque as the agent of choice for lumbar myelography. Water solubility allows free absorption of the material into the blood stream and excretion by the kidneys, as opposed to the uncomfortable and time-consuming manual extraction of oil-based contrast. Furthermore, metrizamide's low viscosity permits the use of a small needle for injection into the subarachnoid space, thus reducing the incidence of spinal headaches resulting from post-puncture leakage. The low iodine content allows greater visibility of the spinal cord, nerves, and other structures. On the other hand, the fact the the metrizamide easily mixes with the spinal fluid makes the examination more difficult because all images must be obtained before the contrast becomes too dilute to be seen.

As a testament to the safety of the metrizamide, there have been no radiographically proven cases of arachnoiditis resulting from the use of this agent. Hansen et al., following the effects of 256 myelograms in 192 patients, found that of the various types of contrast material injected, arachnoiditis developed in 5 of 46 cases after methiodal sodium was used, in 24 of 96 cases using iothalamate meglumine, in 7 of 12 cases using iocarmate meglumine, in 7 of 10 cases using Pantopaque, but in none of 90 cases after metrizamide injection [13].

In its most basic function, myelography is performed to demonstrate localized intradural and extradural masses. Among other indications, the procedure is most effectively utilized when: 1. the clinical signs do not clearly establish the correct level of disc prolapse; 2. prolapse at several levels is suspected; 3. a tumor rather than disc is suspected; 4. cauda equina syndrome is present; 5. lumbar canal stenosis is present; 6. x-rays reveal extensive spondylotic changes [14]. Rothman et al. discusses two primary benefits in the use of myelography [15]. The procedure allows a differentiation of spinal tumors which have been known to mimic symptomatic disc disease during clinical examination, aiding the surgeon in preoperative evaluation. Rothman points out that "several striking examples have been seen in which the history and neurologic findings are characteristic of a herniated lumbar disc at the L4 or L5 level, and yet to the surprise of the treating surgeon, a myelogram revealed a tumor of the lower thoracic or upper lumbar spine." Additionally, the procedure is a useful adjunct to clinical neurological analysis, whereby precise location of nerve root anomalies and disc extrusion as seen on film will help clarify which levels are actually affected. Metrizamide provides an excellent delineation of each spinal nerve subarachnoid extension out into the neural foramina, the cauda equina, as well as more subtle, laterally located spinal lesions. Multiple disc herniations at more than one level are also readily observed. Rothman emphasizes that the neural and anatomic definition permitted by myelography should be fully realized by a complete series of exposures that include anteroposterior, oblique, and standing and prone lateral views.

While this diagnostic tool is extremely helpful and essential as an aid in the preoperative evaluation of a suspected herniation, there is the potential for both false negatives and false positives. Lindsay found that myelograms on asymptomatic individuals will show disc herniation in 10%of patients [16]. A false-negative rate of 16% has been found by Van Damme while DePalma and Rothman have estimated the incidence of overall error in myelography to range from 20% to 30% [5,17]. One explanation for the error rate is that in many situations, a disc prolapse is too small in volume and/or lies too far to the side in the lateral recess of the spinal canal to make significant contact with dural sac [18]. The result is an inability to depict cases of lateral recess stenosis or superior facet entrapment. Camp writes that the expense of myelography (hospitalization required), its failure to diagnose foraminal disease, and the complication rate have rendered it a distant third, where CT and MRI are available [19]. The authors believe that myelography should not be used as a primary factor in deciding whether or not a particular patient should undergo surgical treatment nor should it be used to substantiate or disprove a legal claim in patients who are not surgical candidates. There have been diagnostic problems in which only the myelogram gave the patient a correct diagnosis, even when no surgery was contemplated. Assurance to the patient that the problem was not a malignancy was in and of itself therapeutic.

The diagnostic accuracy of myelography, as demonstrated by surgical observation, is in the range of 75 to 85% [20]. Many reports have compared the efficacy of myelography to computed tomography (CT scan). Voelker et al. evaluated 80 patients with operatively proven lumbar disc herniation or spondyloylysis, and found that metrizamide myelography was accurate in 77% of the cases [20]. Moufarrij et al. found that myelography was predictive of various lumbar pathologies in 83% of 50 patients when confirmed by operative evidence[21]. In a review of 76 patients with surgically confirmed herniated lumbar disc, Bell et al. thought that metrizamide myelography was clearly superior to plain CT (93% accuracy with metrizamide) [22]. Yet Gillstrom et al. examined 90 patients with suspected herniated lumbar discs using myelography and demonstrated that the surgical findings verified 57% of diagnoses, while remarking that CT is as reliable as myelography in the investigation of the lumbar disc herniation [23]. Tchang reached the conclusion that plain CT could replace myelography, based upon his experience with 48 patients with herniated nucleus pulposus [24]. Our experience has shown that imaging techniques can be complimentary. Lateral disc herniations missed on a myelogram may show up on MRI. Clinical correlation is always important in determining the right studies for a given patient.

Computed Axial Tomography (CAT Scan)

The technology of computed axial tomography (CAT scan) was developed in 1973 by Ambrose and Hounsfield. It is a revolutionary, non-invasive method of examining the spinal cord and surrounding structures via a moving x-ray beam arcing around the body. A computer then constructs a picture showing a horizontal cross section of the body that clearly delineates the internal organs, bones, muscles, ligaments and other tissues. Lumbar spine evaluations performed by this technique vary from a series of axial slices to extensive evaluation with multiplanar reconstruction and three-dimensional imaging. Immediately accepted as a cutting-edge diagnostic tool, the inventors of this technology were awarded the Nobel Prize in 1979. That same year, Meyer et al. first reported that herniated lumbar discs could be recognized by CT [25]. The procedure is completely painless to the patient, although a significant amount of radiation is delivered during tomography.

Focus variation of the scanner allows the examination of all structures from dense bone to more lucent fat. More specifically, CT scanning is able to depict associated bony and soft tissue abnormalities, including lateral stenosis, lateral disc herniation, unsuspected bone lesions and facet joint disease. It is the only radiographic modality capable of showing lateral entrapment of the spinal nerve roots by bone and soft tissue. Classic CT findings in the diagnosis of herniated nucleus pulposus follow: a soft tissue mass in the epidural fat, displacement of epidural fat by the posterior disc margin, indentation and compression of the dural sac, compression and displacement of the nerve root sheaths, and calcification or vacuum phenomenon in the disc.

The ability to reconstruct images permits saggital, coronal, oblique and even 3-dimensional visualization of the spine from the initial axial section. Since all reconstruction is executed by computer, no additional radiation or time demands from the patient are necessary. In fact, the total radiation dose delivered with CT scanning is considerably lower than with myelography (6 rads versus 10 rads) [26]. Such features explain why some regard high-quality reformatted spinal CT as the "gold standard" for evaluating complex back injuries. Griebel believes the most significant aspect of CT is that as a non-invasive technique, avoids the infrequent but serious complications associated with myelography, such as post-lumbar puncture headache, infection, arachnoiditis and allergic reaction to contrast material [28]. As a result, the cost and hospitalization associated with myelographic diagnosis can be avoided.

Despite the widely documented success of CT in locating lumbar pathology, the procedure retains some limitations which must be considered. There is some diversity in the accuracy and quality of imaging, depending upon the type of scanner in use. A major problem is the difficulty in distinguishing a bulging annulus from a central disc herniation. As a result of the L3-S1 range generally performed, pathology above L3 will not be detected. Another disadvantage is the identification of post operative epidural scarring, which usually accompanies surgical treatment. As the epidural fat is replaced with fibrotic scar tissue, it becomes increasingly difficult to correctly observe the normal anatomical boundaries. The implication is that a CT scan of those patients who have had lumbar surgery must often be supplemented by some other test, such as myelography or MRI.

The inability to distinguish between the herniated disc and the dural sac is another limitation that can result if there is a large or small herniated disc in patients with little or no epidural fat, particularly in subjects with spinal stenosis and a decrease in the amount of cerebrospinal fluid. According to Camp, the primary limitation of CT is its consistent inability to show intrathecal pathology, compared to MRI [19]. However, visibility of the lumbar area has been significantly improved with the intrathecal injection of metrizamide preceding scanning, known as contrast-enhanced CT scanning. Unlike non-contrast CT, metrizamide scanning provides greater clarity of the dural sac, spinal cord and nerve roots, the result of differences in density between the contrast material and adjacent soft tissues.

CT scanning has proven to be very accurate in its depiction of the herniated nucleus pulposus, which the scan shows as a posterior or posterolateral extension of the disc margin with displacement of the epidural fat, deformity of the dural sac and dislocation of the root sleeves [26]. The disc size and level can be accurately determined preoperatively. Some cases of laterally herniated discs show a cork-like lesion completely filling the corresponding neural foramen and obliterating the epidural fat, compressing the corresponding nerve root. Correct diagnosis of lumbar disc herniation using CT has been shown in the literature to range from 72% to 100%. Griebel et al. followed 100 consecutive patients with suspected lumbar disc herniation pre- and postoperatively, using CT to clarify the nature of sciatica and low back pain [26]. While a herniated lumbar disc was found at surgery in 96 of 100 of the patients, CT revealed disc pathology in 94 of the 100. This compares with the lower rate of accuracy for myelograms, where 74 of the 86 patients studied by myelogram demonstrated a disc pathology confirmed by surgical observation.

Moufarrij confirmed that CT is highly predictive of surgical findings, but only for a very specific group of patients [27]. Careful selection of 50 patients presenting with sciatica and suspected lumbar disc herniation was completed in an effort to screen out those patients with a history of prior lumbar laminectomy (one of the limitations of CT noted earlier) or a clinical diagnosis of lumbar canal stenosis. Each of the 50 participants was studied by CT scan, while a myelogram was administered to 46 of the patients. The results of the scanning were broken down into five groups, according to the pathology diagnosed by CT: soft herniated disc, spondylitic compression, spondylosis and disc protrusion, negative CT scan, and sacral nerve root cyst. The accuracy of CT was shown to vary greatly with the nature of the pathology, and in only one group was CT judged more effective than myelography.

The best CT results were found in the group diagnosed with soft herniation, where CT correctly predicted the pathological condition in the 21 patients with disc protrusion as the only operative finding and partially predicted the condition in 3 of the patients, thus verifying protrusion in 24 of 25 patients (96%). The 10 patients predicted as having spondylitic compression were all incompletely diagnosed by CT. Most of these patients had disc protrusion in addition to spondylitic compression. In the group diagnosed with spondylosis and disc protrusion, CT was only partially correct in diagnosing 3 patients and fully correct in one of the four patients.

CT performed much worse in the group of patients initially diagnosed with negative signs; of the ten patients in that group, CT was incorrect in nine of the cases, all of whom had definite findings at operation, while one patient did indeed show no pathology at surgery. It was in this CT negative group that myelography was clearly more predictive of surgical findings, demonstrating disc protrusion in seven patients. As for the one patient presenting with a suspected sacral nerve root cyst, CT was correct in its prediction of an extradural lesion. The cumulative success rate of CT in all five categories was found to be completely correct in 48%, partially correct in 24% and incorrect in 28%. Thus, the 72% of cases in which CT either partially or completely predicted pathology is significantly less than number of patients (83%) correctly diagnosed by myelography.

The most significant finding of the study was the 96% successful rate of prediction in patients with disc protrusion as the only CT finding. This can be favorably compared to a number of other reports which demonstrate similarly high rates of correct diagnosis. Carrera et al. reported 28 disc protrusions found at operation out of 29 disc protrusions predicted by CT, while Benjamin found a concurrence rate of 100% among 38 predicted disc protrusions confirmed by surgery [28,29]. Haugton et al. reported a CT prediction rate of 29 out of 30 disc protrusion verified post-operatively [30]. The same study also found that CT was incorrectly interpreted in 6 of 11 patients with spondylosis or a bulging annulus. This correlates strongly with the results of the Moufarrij report, which documented the apparent inability of CT to diagnose patients with such pathology. The high number of false-negative scans is also noteworthy, with 9 of 50 patients unable to be diagnosed properly by the CT. If anything, this ratio indicates the necessity of utilizing other imaging tools in the evaluation of lumbar pathology, particularly in the event of a negative CT scan on a symptomatic patient.

As in the above study by Moufarrij, the use of CT in conjunction with myelography will improve the accuracy of diagnosis in most cases. Using metrizamide-enhanced CT as an adjunct to metrizamide myelography, Voelker et al. examined the predictive accuracy of the two techniques in eighty patients with operatively proven lumbar disc herniation or spondylosis, and found results which support such a conclusion [20]. Of the 42 patients presenting with operatively-confirmed disc extrusion, the enhanced CT was was correct in 81% of the cases, while myelography was positive in 79%. Cumulatively, 4 out of 42 discs were not observed, resulting in an overall accuracy rate of 90%. In the examination of 46 patients with confirmed spondylosis, CT was predictive in 83%, myleography in 76% and the combination of techniques were diagnostic in 91% of the cases. Taking all of the cases together, there was an increase in the percentage of cases diagnosed by both techniques over those diagnosed individually by either metrizamide-enhanced CT or metrizamide myelography. Furthermore, it was found that among the misdiagnosed cases, spinal stenosis and postoperative epidural scarring was a primary factor in diagnostic failure, even if both tests were performed.

The following summarized data from the Whitman Institute of Neuroscience clearly indicates that the most economical diagnostic test for low back injury is not always the least expensive [19]. Rather, it is the one that most often yields the complete and correct diagnosis. A total of 222 consecutive patients charged for conventional CT only, myelography only, and both tests combined were reviewed. This last combination is significant, due to the fact that the use of conventional CT or myelograpy yielded sufficient clinical uncertainty to require both exams in 22% of the patients in the series. The average charge per patient was calculated as follows: – CT only -- $375.00; Myelography only – $1780.00; CT and Myelography – $2240.00. In a similar analysis of 508 patients, the cost of diagnosis using the most accurate CT imaging (with multiplanar reformatting) compared with myelography was: CT/MPR – $654.00; Myelography – $1,791.00; Myelography and CT/MPR – $2,434.00.

Based upon cost calculations, it was concluded that the reformatted CT scan gave the most informative and economical diagnosis in the vast majority of cases. While axial CT scanning was the least expensive single test, the lack of unequivocal information required supplementary myelographic data, dramatically increasing the cost. Regardless of how much information myelography provides, the significant costs of hospitalization and occasional complications resulted in an average cost over twice that of reformatted CT and nearly five times the cost of axial CT.

Magnetic Resonance Imaging

Magnetic resonance imaging (MRI) is the current state-of-the-art in computer-aided imaging technology. The first magnetic resonance images of humans were produced in 1977 [31]. The test is completely non-invasive, does not require the use of ionizing radiation and has no known adverse effects. It yields excellent resolution of soft tissues, and is of particular value in visualizing the lumbar spine and its neural contents. Providing information about the anatomic relationships of the spinal canal, vertebral bodies and intervertebral disc material, numerous studies have shown MRI to have equal or greater specificity (ability to identify those individuals free of a condition) and sensitivity (ability to correctly identify those with a condition) than CT scan and myelography. The remainder of this section will compare the efficacy of MRI to other diagnostic modalities, including CT, myelography and discography, detailing what the distinct advantages and disadvantages of MRI are.

MRI employs a powerful magnetic field to produce a uniform alignment of hydrogen atom protons (nuclei) in the body. Radio signals generated from the tissues are reassembled into a visual images. The strength of the radio signal that is received from a given tissue will depend on the number of hydrogen protons and how mobile they are. The images are displayed in varying intensities of a grey scale. For example, fat is displayed as bright (high signal intensity), muscle has an intermediate signal intensity, and cortical bone, low in hydrogen content, cannot be readily observed. This is definitely not the case with the disc, as a depiction of herniation is clearly observed. The chemical makeup of the disc allows MRI to distinguish the nucleus pulposus from the annulus fibrosus, thereby indicating a prolapse of nuclear material through the annular fibers. Additionally, many of the same spinal pathologies seen with conventional radiography, myelography and CT are also demonstrated using MRI – including intervertebral disc space narrowing, disk bulges, spondylolisthesis and osteophyte formation.

MRI provides several distinct advantages over CT, the diagnostic modality previously thought to be the technique of choice in the evaluation of lumbar abnormalities. While the spatial resolution of axial CT currently exceeds that of axial MRI, the soft tissue contrast resolution of MRI is superior to that of CT. Contrast can be easily varied by changing the pulse sequence of the machine to match the molecular composition of specific sites of patholgy. MRI quite distinctively identifies fat, cerebrospinal fluid, nerve roots, fibrotic tissue, fibrosus of the annulus and both a normal and abnormal nucleus pulposus [31]. MRI is capable of indicating degenerative changes in the disc before there are gross anatomical changes. Because the test is completely non-invasive and free of ionizing radiation, one is safely able to repeat examinations with MRI frequently to follow-up on treatment and track disease progress.

MRI can also provide more information than CT by directly imaging large regions of the spine in sagittal, axial and coronal planes while maintaining high image quality, while CT is able to examine the spine in the direct axial plane only [32]. This becomes an invaluable aid in excluding the combination of symptomatic disc and asymptomatic tumor. Lastly, the absence of bone artifacts with MRI is an important advantage over CT in the investigation of the spinal canal. The limitations of MRI include: the inability to demonstrate calcification of cortical bone, the difficulty of investigating the very sick or uncooperative patient, the high cost of the equipment and support structure (as much as $3 million) and consequently high treatment costs, and slow patient throughput [33]. Moreover, some MRI instruments miss subtle disc abnormalities due to an inability to produce slices narrow enough prevent a gap of 3-4mm between adjacent images.

Currently, the most important application of MRI in the lumbar area is the evaluation of intervertebral disc diseases. Only MRI has demonstrated promise in depicting early changes of disc degeneration through non-invasive means. Since the MRI demonstrates a uniformly bright magnetic signal intensity in the discs of a normal spine with no posterior bulging, a slight attenuation in brilliance is interpreted as mild degeneration. The images of the disc and nucleus are particularly clear when T2-weighted imaging sequences are used.

A realistic example of the applications of MRI to analysis of disc degeneration is reported by Gibson et al. in the imaging of adolescent disc herniation [34]. A comparison of the MRI appearance of the spine was made between 20 adolescents (age range between 14 and 19 years) with proven symptomatic disc herniations and a control group of 20 asymptomatic patients. Results of the study supported the very strong correlation between magnetic signal weakness and intervertebral nuclear degeneration/prolapse. The MRI scans indicated abnormal discs in all of the 20 patients with proven or symptomatic disc herniation, all of which were detected by a reduction in the intensity of the signal from the nucleus pulposus on the parasagittal and sagittal sections. The abnormal disc was always present at the same level diagnosed by other clinical examinations, where varying degrees of posterior nuclear protrusion were observed at the same site. An irregularity in the normally smooth nucleus outline was also noted in this group of patients. As for the asymptomatic subjects, the MRI scans found evidence of disc abnormality in 4 of the 20 control patients, three of which were found to have a single-level pathology compatible with minor central disc protrusions.

Gibson concludes: "The reduction in the signal from the nucleus pulposus was an example of the unique information provided by MRI on the 'state of health' of the intervertebral disc. The high signal from the nucleus pulposus on T2-weighted images probably reflects the high nuclear-water content of normal intervertebral discs. It has been shown that within a few hours of a disc herniation, the water content of the nucleus pulposus falls by at least 10% and although it increases again later, it never returns to normal. It is probably this change in water content that produces the reduction in the intensity of the MRI signal from the nucleus pulposus of a herniated disc."

In another study, Schneiderman et al. evaluated 101 disc levels among 36 patients with low back pain in an effort to analyze the effects of aging on nuclear water content as depicted by MRI scan [35]. It was found that normal disc signal intensity on MRI indicated normal morpholgy in all the patients with symptoms greater than two months. In 100 of 101 disc levels evaluated, an abnormal disc signal intensity was correlated with degenerative changes seen on discography. Significantly, the exact pattern of the degenerative changes could not be predicted on signal intensity alone. Schneiderman remarks: "Changes in intervertebral disc signal strength seen on MRI accurately reflect the presence or absence of degenerative changes seen on discography in patients with low back pain... Discography is not indicated when MRI demonstrates normal disc intensity. Clinically, MRI is helpful in assessing the affected disc level as well as the adjacent disc levels in patients with low-back pain and spondylolisthesis."

Other Techniques

Thermography

Thermography is a relatively new diagnostic technique that provides information on soft tissue injury and disc pathology. The test is totally non-invasive, does not require hospitalization or use of ionizing radiation, and has no known side-effects. Thermography measures local skin temperature, providing physiological information mediated through the autonomic nerve fibers. Extensive research of body dermatomes and myotomes has indicated that temperature patterns from homologous sides of the body are remarkably constant within a narrow range of temperature.

Symmetric heat emission from the extremities is the foundation for thermographic investigation of suspected nerve root lesions. Temperature differences between the normal side and the affected side must be consistent in order to show pathology. As a rule, the tissue in distress generates heat radiation which can be seen and imaged for qualitative and quantitative interpretation via thermography. For example, S1 root involvement may be associated with localized increased heat emission from the affected side of the lumbosacral region (specifically the ipsilateral posterior thigh, and posterior and lateral aspects of the leg). L5 root involvement may be characterized by abnormal heat emission of the ipsilateral midgluteal region, lateral thigh and anterior leg. Root pathology at L4 may involve abnormal heat emission of the ipsilateral anterior thigh, and medial aspects of the leg and ankle.

Although there are frequent minor variations and nerve fiber crossovers, temperature fluctuations at particular dermatomes and myotomes reflect dysfunction in root compression syndromes. Thus, an abnormal thermogram may be a useful indicator of nerve root irritation, peripheral nerve injury or vertebral soft tissue damage caused by a variety of disorders, including intervertebral disc bulging and prolapse. A majority of the literature has reported a high correlation between positive thermographic findings and pain in many lumbar disorders, as well as a high consistency with other positive diagnostic tests such as CT scan and myelography.

A comparison between thermography and MRI is reported by Goldberg in a retrospective evaluation of 31 low-back patients [36]. Eight of these patients were also administered myelograms. A very strong correlation between myelography, MRI and thermography was observed. In those cases when thermography was negative, no grossly abnormal MRI scans or myelograms were found. When the thermogram presented definite positive evidence of disc pathology, MRI revealed only 69% of those patients, the remaining 31% judged were as either minimal or normal findings. Goldberg relates the difference to the percentage of laterally protruding abnormal discs and certain arthritic spurs of cortical bone not easily visualized with MRI. It was also observed that there were no false negative nor false positive interpretations found when thermography was compared to myelography. Goldberg is careful to note that since false positive evaluations do occur with thermographic evaluations (as well as CT scan and myelography), all such positive findings must be carefully correlated with the clinical findings in each individual patient.

The predictive accuracy of thermography was evaluated in a more rigorous study by Weinstein [37]. The results obtained from thermographic evaluation of 500 patients with complaints of lumbar back pain were compared to four alternative diagnostic modalities: EMG, CT scanning, myelography and surgical exploration. The thermogram agreed with the EMG evaluation in 80% of the cases (68/80) when both tests were positive and 100% (76/76) when both tests were negative, yielding an overall concurrence rate of 92%. With regard to the CT scan, thermography correlated with 83% of the patients receiving both procedures (171/206), and an overall accuracy rate of 90% was observed (based upon diagnosis with both modalities). Compared with myelography, the two tests agreed in 70% of patients (38/54), leading to an overall rate of 91% predictive accuracy. A concurrence of 100% was observed in 34 patients undergoing both surgical exploration and thermography. The cumulative total rate of agreement between thermography and all four modalities was calculated to be 86% (387/450). Among the 63 instances in which a comparative test disagreed, 34 of the positive thermograms were confirmed by an alternative diagnostic procedure, thereby providing an overall accuracy rate of 93.6%.

Perhaps the most notable finding in this comparative study was that of the 134 negative thermograms, only one false negative test was found, resulting in a concurrence rate of 99% with alternative diagnostic testing. As for the positive thermograms, the test remained approximately 10% more accurate than EMG testing and CT scanning, and an impressive 22% higher than myelography. Weinstein concludes: "The primary value of the study is its documentation suggesting the concept that a negative thermogram will almost inevitably be confirmed by a corresponding negative test, regardless of the test used. This finding suggests the recognition of thermography as one of the valuable tools available to clinicians. This fact alone places the thermogram firmly into the diagnostic armamentarium as a valuable and cost-effective modality."

Yet another enthusiastic endorsement of the procedure is seen in a study by Pochaczevsky [38]. Liquid-crystal contact thermography was performed on 101 patients complaining of lumbar and sciatic pain, 61 of whom had already undergone myelographic and clinical examination. Of these 61 subjects, 79% had a positive thermogram, while 62% presented positive myelography. Twenty-three patients had negative or questionable myelograms. Surgical observation was able to confirm the results in 38 patients, indicating that the overall accuracy of thermography was 95%, compared with 84% for myelography (all figures based upon completely surgically proven results). As in the other two studies listed above, thermography showed no false-negative evidence, whereas myelography was equivocal or falsely-negative in six patients.

Other studies have reported similarly high rates of surgically-confirmed accuracy. In a review of 24 patients presenting operative findings of herniated disc, Raskin et al. concluded that thermography was accurate in 71% of the series39. Edeiken et al. found thermography to be accurate in predicting disc herniation in 80% of 29 surgical cases [40]. Wexler found that thermography of the spine and extremities was 92% accurate when compared to the physical findings of 86 patients [41]. While all of the preceding studies firmly embrace thermography as a highly diagnostic tool, a 1988 survey of 293 orthopedic surgeons by Ash & Foster suggests otherwise [42]. Only 7 surgeons reported finding thermography helpful in the diagnosis of neck and low back pain. The authors concluded that this study did not support the use of thermography in the courtroom to document painful conditions of the neck and back.

A number of significant findings emerge from the preceding discussion of current literature regarding the usefulness of thermography as competently summarized by Pochaczevsky: "Since thermography is a non-invasive technique that appears to be highly sensitive, it may play an important role in selecting those patients who require myelography, thereby improving the efficacy of the latter study. In the appropriate clinical setting, a negative thermogram may therefore obviate a myelogram. It may also be valuable in the evaluation of patients with negative or questionable myelograms. Thermography may further complement myelography in helping to determine which abnormalities are clinically significant. Thermography helps confirm clinically suspected spinal root compression syndromes, as seen in association with herniated disks and osteophyte formation, spinal canal stenosis including lateral recess stenosis, and subluxation and hypertrophy of superior vertebral facets. It graphically documents pain in spinal musculoligamentous injuries even when roentgenographic studies are normal... It identifies and graphically demonstrates otherwise purely subjective pain patterns and helps document and distinguish true somatic complaints from malingering." In contrast, Frymoyer states that "thermography has little value in evaluating the cause of a patient's low back pain" [43].

Electromyography (EMG)

EMG testing is based upon the electrical activity of nerves and muscles. The electrical properties of tissue were first described by Luigi Galvani in the late 18th century. In 1929 Adrion and Bonk developed the concentric needle electrode which permitted accurate measurement of voltage deep within living human muscle tissue. On this foundation the modern science of electromyography has been built [44].

In low back pain EMG is useful when the clinical examination is confusing. A positive EMG suggests structural as opposed to functional pathology [45]. Clinical electromyography requires great skill and judgement. Undue confidence in equivocal or non-diagnostic abnormalities can lead to frequent false positive results46. In addition to concentric needle voltage recording, surface recording of muscle activity is possible. Cram et al. used such surface recording to study the postural component of chronic low back pain[47].

Fifty subjects were selected, 80% of whom had low back pain as their primary complaint. The patients were then monitored by surface EMGs in both the sitting and standing positions. The results indicated a higher than normal EMG level for standing in the chronic low back patients. The mean level of bilateral EMG activity was not found to be a significant predictor of those with low back pain. However, the asymmetrical EMG evaluation provided differentiation for the low back group. A statistically significant imbalance in EMG activity was observed in the right versus left lumbar and cervical paraspinalis. Cram's study suggests that posture or position (sitting versus standing) can significantly alter surface EMG findings, particularly for the lumbar paraspinalis and abdominal muscle group. "It appears that, as the patient with low back pain shifts weight to one side in a 'protective guarding' manner, an imbalance in the EMG levels between the right and left lumbar paraspinals would result. In addition the patient might shift the position of the head to the right or left for gravitational balance, generating an additional imbalance between the right and left cervical paraspinalis EMG levels."

Such a conclusion is consistent with the theory that EMG levels among chronic low back patients will be abnormal. The theory holds that back sufferers will have higher levels of paraspinal muscle activity during rest and movement when compared to individuals without chronic low back pain. Yet this concept is challenged by Collins et al, who have demonstrated that chronic low back pain does not automatically cause overexertion of the lumbar muscle tissue [48]. Their report is based on a study of eleven chronic low back patients exposed to different postures and stresses designed to activate the back muscles. It was found that this group exhibited similar or significantly less paraspinal muscle activity than an age-matched control group. In addition, there were no significant differences in left-right paraspinal muscle activity between the two groups. A similar finding was reported by Ahern et al., where the average EMG levels during static and postural movement showed no statistically significant difference between 40 surgical and 30 nonsurgical patients [49].

The primary disadvantage of EMG is the limited information it can offer regarding the etiology of low back pain. Even when the EMG is abnormal, precise interspace localization can never be as definite as demonstrated by imaging methods, owing to anatomic variation in muscle innervation and nerve roots. By the same token, a normal EMG would tend to exclude significant constant neuropathic disorder at any level, but need not rule out ligamentous, muscular, osseous, or intermittent cause of pain. Furthermore, the procedure of attaching electrodes to muscle tissue can be unpleasant and painful. Patients with severe pain, low pain thresholds, excessive anxiety or conflicting emotional symptoms may not be able to participate fully in the examination, resulting in an inconclusive study [44].

Discography

Lumbar discography is perhaps the most controversial modality used in the investigation of intervertebral disc degeneration. Discography involves the injection of imaging material directly into the nucleus pulposus of the disc. Information is then recorded about the amount of dye accepted, the pressure necessary to inject the material, the configuration of the opaque material, and the reproduction of the patient's pain. The objective is twofold: to radiographically visualize the extent of disc damage, and to provoke a painful response which the patient can compare with the primary clinical complaint. The reader will recall from the chapter on etilogy that the injection of non-reactive saline solution into the disc can produce a radiating pain in the back, buttock and upper thigh. Given the obscure nature of lumbar pain, a reproduction of the precise pain experienced by the patient is considered to be of immeasurable value in the localization of pathology. However, a complete dichotomy of opinion is observed in the literature over the significance and validity of any objective evidence derived from discography.

On one side are the proponents who strongly believe in the mechanics of discography. A primary part of the logic of the procedure is concerned with the volume of liquid the disc is able to contain upon injection. Bernard argues that the normal lumbar disk accepts between 0.5 and 1.5 ml of contrast solution with firm resistance during injection, while an abnormal disc will accept significantly more volume without resistance [50]. The advocates of discography consider a symptomatic degenerative disc to be one that disperses injected contrast in all directions, extending to the outer margins of the annulus and possibly into epidural space as well. Simultaneously, a painful reaction is provoked in the patient that will, under ideal circumstances, reproduce the patient's current pain complex.

Significantly, much of literature that supports the use of discography tends to dismiss the importance of radiographic imaging. Instead, many feel that "the subjective perception of pain by the patient during the procedure is often more important to the clinician than the pattern produced by the intradiscal injection of contrast medium" [51]. Discography is also credited with the clarification of ambiguous findings from CT and MRI, two modalities which can only reveal a static picture of the lumbar disk, frequently displaying evidence of questionable clinical significance, such as a "bulging disk". Discography is a useful tool in assessing whether such a disk is actually symptomatic, acting as confirmation of the original diagnosis. False negative discograms are reported not to occur, and therefore are capable of establishing that a disc is normal. Provocation of pain is argued to be the only method of confirming multiple level disc pathologies. Thus, when other diagnostic tests have indicated surgical correction is needed, discography allows the surgeon to choose which levels should be included in a surgical procedure [51].

All of this is dismissed as rubbish by the opponents of the technique. One disillusioned researcher relegated discography to the "Hall of Fame of Bygone Radiologic Techniques" [52]. Scullin claims that the procedure is the only imaging test that shows positive results despite normal findings by CT scan and metrizamide myelography, adding that many doctors perform surgery "based on the results of a test that... is considered invalid by the overwhelming majority of academic radiologists in this country" [53]. The notion that leakage of contrast material through the annulus necessitates surgery is critically questioned. The opponents believe there is no possible way for a radiologist to differentiate an annular fissure from a tear when leakage does occur, let alone make a judgement call for surgery in spite of negative CT or myelographic exploration. Recognition of the temptation to operate by enthusiastic surgeons prompts Weisel to remark: "The test is often misused in symptomatic patients without objective findings as a last resort for pseudo-justification for surgical intervention for psychogenic backache" [54]. The pain-producing capability of disc injection is also hotly contested, opponents pointing to the high probability of pain being experienced at one of the three lowest lumbar levels, even if the patient is asymptomatic and the disc is normal. Additionally, no research has reliably determined that the needle puncture and injection of contrast material into the disc will not encourage disk degeneration and herniation.

How does discography compare with other radiographic techniques in diagnostic accuracy? A report by Grubb et al. evaluated the value of lumbar roentgenograms, metrizamide myelography and discography in an identification of the structural sources of low back pain [55]. Selected for analysis was 108 patients with chronic low back pain, nearly all of whom complained of both back and leg pain. On account of their symptoms, 77% of the patients considered themselves unable to continue with their normal jobs. While all of the patients had had previous roentgenograms and 60% had had myelography, none had been evaluated using discography.

The results of the study found the diagnostic value of discography to be quite consistent. Discography was performed on a total of 346 discs, an average of 3 discs per patient. The majority of the normal discs were nonpainful (88%), except when adjacent to a painful abnormal disc or in patients with significant psychological or extra-spinal pathology. The majority of the abnormal discs were painful (78%). Of the discs identified as abnormal by discography, only 38.5% were identified as abnormal by roentgenograms and only 31% were identified as abnormal by myelography. Correct identification of abnormal disc levels occurred in only 36% of the patients. Roentgenographic and myelographic findings were frequently absent at discs that caused a reproduction of the patients usual pain on discography.

Discography has been shown to correlate very consistently with findings of disc degeneration by MRI, discussed above in the Schneiderman report[35]. The article presented convincing evidence which enthusiastically validated the accuracy of MRI, indicated by the 99% concurrence rate in predicting abnormality or normality as determined by discography. While such accuracy is truly impressive, the use of discography is by no means rejected in favor of MRI. The investigators had this to say about the efficacy of discography: "Discography still has its place in the diagnostic acumen. If a disc is degenerative and fusion is being considered, discography may provide information as to the symptomatic nature of this disc level. We think that reproduction of pain with discography is helpful in the assessment of these abnormal disc levels. In the presence of decreased signal intensity on MRI, we might still proceed with discography. However, discography is not indicated when MRI demonstrates normal disc intensity."

The application of discography in the preoperative examination of fusion candidates is thought by one advocate to be the principle benefit of discal injection [55]. For instance, it was reported that discography was responsible for an improvement in the clinical results of some 350 patients undergoing spinal fusion for scoliosis [56]. Before discography was used to help determine which levels should be included in fusion, the success rate of pain relief after fusion was 67%, which rose to 85% after discography was adapted to the diagnostic procedure. The logic of the argument favoring the technique is illustrated by the following quotation: "Discography is not a test that when positive, points the surgeon to surgery. Rather, when other diagnostic tests or diagnoses have indicated surgical correction is needed, discography allows the surgeon to choose which levels should be included in a surgical procedure."

Bone Scanning

Bone scanning is a procedure in which radioactive bone-seeking compounds are injected intravenously, attracted to metabolically active bone and joint locations. Detectors show the areas of radioactive uptake, which reveal areas of bone activity and new bone growth. The most commonly used agent is Technetium. Also known as radionuclide imaging, the technique may be more sensitive than radiography in detecting metastasis, Paget's disease, inflammatory conditions such as ankylosing spondylitis, spondylolysis, sacroiliitis, subtle trauma, and certain specific tumors such as osteoid osteoma [57]. Berg considers bone scans to be far more sensitive than normal radiography in the detection of early bone lesions because nearly 50% destruction of cancellous bone is needed before a lytic process is apparent on plain film [3]. Furthermore, he suggests that "bone scans should replace radiographs as the primary study in almost all cases of suspected metastatic disease and totally in most cases of suspected primary neoplasm."

Whether or not radionuclide bone scans can be effectively applied to the diagnosis of lumbar disc degeneration is debatable. It is hypothesized that disc and vertebral body degeneration create a level of inflammation that might attract enough imaging material, thereby providing information about the patholgy. The theory was not confirmed by Johanssen et al. in their attempt to locate the level of myelographically confirmed lumbar disc herniation via bone scan [58]. In none of the ten patients could accumulation of radioactivity (using Technetium) in the bony structures of the affected lumbar segment be demonstrated.

Additional evidence demonstrates that the real diagnostic strength of bone scanning is not with the generic low back case, but rather with the low-back patient presenting with a known malignancy. Schutte et al. studied the results of bone scanning on a group of 38 patients suffering "non-specific" back pain (no disease recognized), and a second group of 138 presenting with back pain and a known malignant disease [57]. It was observed that 81.5% of the group with "non-specific" back pain had a negative bone scan; significantly, every patient that tested positive also had an elevated erythrocyte sedimentation rate. Out of the 138 cancer patients, 40% presented a positive scan attributed to metastasis. This can be compared to the findings of Schaffer et al., which reported that where bone pain was noted, the association between a positive bone scan and the presence of bone metastasis was 60% [59]. Schutte concludes: "The present findings indicate that bone scintigraphy is not a useful procedure in patients with long-standing low back pain who have normal radiographs and normal laboratory findings."

References

1. McCall IW, Butt WP: The radiological diagnosis of low back pain. Current Orthop 1:375-382, 1987.
2. Thomas JC, Jr. From Watkins RG, Collis JS, Jr. (Eds.): Lumbar discectomy and laminectomy - Priniciples and techniques in spine surgery. Aspen, 1987, pp. 45-50.
3. Berg D: The radiologic evaluation of back pain. From Low Back Pain (Stanton-Hicks, Boas - Eds). Raven Press, New York 1982.
4. Roberts F, Keshore P, Cunningham N: Routine oblique radiography of the pediatric lumbar spine: Is it necessary? AJR 131:297-298, 1978.

5. Van Damme W, Hessels G, Verhelst M, Van Laer L, Van Es I: Relative efficacy of clinical examination, electromyography, plain films radiography, myelography and lumbar phebography in the diagnosis of low back pain and sciatica. Neuroradiology 18:109-118, 1979.
6. Splithoff C: Lumbosacral Junction – Roentgenographic comparison of patients with and without backaches. JAMA (August 22, 1953) Pgs 1610-1613.
7. Barton PN, Biram JH: Pre-placement x-ray examination of the lower back. Industr Med 15:319, 1946.
8. Witt I, Vestergaard A, Rosenklint A: A comparative analysis of x-ray findings of the lumbar spine in patients with and without lumbar pain. Spine 9:298-300, 1984.
9. Bailey W: Observation on the etiology and frequency of spondylolisthesis and its precursors. Radiology 48:107-112, 1947.
10. Friedman MM, Fischer FJ, Van Demark RF: Lumbosacral roentgenograms of 100 soldiers; Control study. Amer J Roentgenol & Rad Therapy 55:292-298, 1946.
11. Nachemson A: The Lumbar Spine - An Orthopedic Challenge. Spine 1:59-71, 1976.
12. Frymoyer JW, Phillips RB, Newberg AH, MacPherson BV: A comparative analysis of the interpretations of lumbar spinal radiographs by chiropractors and medical doctors. Spine 11:1020-1023, 1986.
13. Hansen EB, Fahrenkrug A, Praestholm J: Late memingeal effects of myelographic contrast media with special reference of metrizamide. Br J of Radiology 51:321-327, 1978.
14. Ramani PS: Low back pain and sciatica. Quarterly Medical Review 33:1-26, 1982.
15. Rothman RH, Simeone FA: The Spine. 2nd Edition WB Saunders, Philadelphia, 1982,
16. Lindsay ELS: Incidental lumbo-sacral myelographic abnormalities shown by water soluble contrast medium. Clin Radiol 36:647-649, 1985.
17. DePalma AF, Rothman RH: The intervertebral disc. W.B. Saunders, Philadelphia, 1970, pp. 241-247.
18. Epstein JA, Epstein BS, Rosenthal AD, et al.: Sciatica caused by nerve root entrapment in the lateral recess: The superior facet syndrome. J Neurosurg 36:584-589, 1972.
19. Camp PE: Invasive procedures for treating herniated discs: Clinical and cost considerations. Occup Med: State of the Art Reviews 3(1):75-90, 1988.
20. Voelker JL, Mealey J, Eskridge JM, Gilmor RL: Metrizamide-enhanced computed tomography as an adjunct to metrizamide myelography in the evaluation of lumbar disc herniation and spondylosis. Neurosurg 20:379-384, 1987.

21. Moufarrij NA, Hardy RW, Weinstein MA: Computed tomographic, myelographic, and operative findings in patients with suspected herniated lumbar discs. Neurosurgery 12:184-188, 1983.
22. Bell GR, Rothman RH, Booth RE, Cuckler JM, Garfin S, Herkowitz H, Simeone FA, Dolinskas C, Han SS: A study of computer-assisted tomography: II. Comparison of metrizamide myelography and computed tomography in the diagnosis of herniated lumbar disc and spinal stenosis. Spine 9:552-556, 1984.
23. Gillstrom P, Ericsson K, Hindmarsh T: A comparison of computed tomography and myelography in the diagnosis of lumbar disc herniation. Arch Orthop Trauma Surg 106:12-14, 1986.
24. Tchang SPK, Howie JL, Kirkaldy-Willis WH, Paine KWE, Moola D: Computed tomography versus myelography in diagnosis of lumbar disc herniation. J Can Assoc Radiol 33:15-20, 1982.
25. Meyer GA, Haughton VM, Williams AL: Diagnosis of herniated lumbar disc with computed tomography. N Engl J Med 301:1166-1167, 1979.
26. Griebel R, Tchang S, Khan M, Varughese G: Correlation of computed tomography with surgical diagnosis in lumbar disc disease. Can J Neurol Sciences 10:248-251, 1983.
27. Carrera GF, Williams AL, Haughton VM: Computed tomography in sciatica. Radiology 137:433-437, 1980.
28. Benjamin V, Mangiardi JR, Lin J, Baun I: The value of CT versus conventional myelography inthe diagnosis and surgical treatment of lumbar disc disease. Presented at the 51st Annual Meeting of the American Association of Neurological Surgeons, Honolulu, Hawaii, April 27, 1982.
29. Haughton VM, Eldevik OP, Magnaes B, Amundsen P: A prospective comparison of computed tomography and myelography in the diagnosis of herniated lumbar disc. Radiology 142:103-10, 1982.
30. Hinshaw WS, Bottomley PA, Holland GN: Radiographic thin section image of the human wrist by nuclear magnetic resonance. Nature 270:722-723, 1977.
31. Weisz GM, Kitchener PN: The use of magnetic resonance imaging in the diagnosis of postoperative lumbar conditions. Med J of Austr 146: 99-101, 1987.
32. Richardson ML, Genant HK, Helms CA, Gillespy T, Heller M, Jergesen HE, Bovill EG: Magnetic resonance imaging of the musculoskeletal system. Synposium on Computed Tomography. Orthop Clin North Am 16(3):569-87, 1985.
33. Steiner RE: Magnetic resonance imaging — its impact on diagnostic radiology. Caldwell Lecture. AJR 145:883-889, 1985.
34. Gibson MJ, Szypryt EP, Buckley JH, Worthington BS, Mulholland RC: Magnetic resonance imaging of adolescent disc herniation. J Bone Joint Surgery 69B:699-703, 1987.

35. Schneiderman G, Flannigan B, Kingston S, Thomas J, Dillin WH, Watkins RG: Magnetic resonance imaging in the diagnosis of disc degeneration: Correlation with discography. Spine 12(3):276-81, 1987.
36. Goldberg GS: Thermography and MRI correlated in 31 cases. PostGradMar(54-8), 1986.
37. Weinstein SA, Weinstein G: A review of 500 patients with low back complaints: Comparison of five clinically-accepted diagnostic modalities. Post Grad Med, Mar 1986, Spec 40-3.
38. Pochaczevsky R, Wexler CE, Meyers PH, Epstein JA, Marc JA: Thermographic study of extremity dermatomes in the diagnosis of spinal root compression syndromes. Biomed Therm (1982):339-360.
39. Raskin MR, Martin-Lopez M, Sheldon JJ: Lumbar thermography in discogenic diseases. Radiology 119:149-152, 1976.
40. Edeiken J, Wallace JD, Curley RF, et al: Thermography and herniated lumbar disks. Am J Roentgenol 102:790-796, 1968.
41. Wexler CE: Thermographic evaluation of trauma (spine). Acta Thermograph 5:3-11, 1980.
42. Ash CJ, Foster MV: Neuromuscular thermography in orthopedic surgery - a usage poll. Orthop Rev 6:589-92, 1988.
43. Frymoyer JW: Occupational Low Back Pain. Praeger Scientific, 1984, p. 178.
44. Green L: Electrodiagnostic studies in low back pain. Part II. From Finneson BE: Low Back Pain. JB Lipincott, Philadelphia, 1980. pp 58-60.
45. Seimon LP: Low back pain. Clinical Diagnosis and Management. Appleton-Century-Crofts, 1983. pp. 51, 62.
46. Kirkaldy-Willis WH: Managing Low Back Pain. Churchill Livingstone, 1988, p. 163.
47. Cram JR, Steger JC: EMG scanning in the diagnosis of chronic pain. Biofeedback and Self-Regulation 8:229-241, 1983.
48. Collins GA, Cohen MJ, Naliboff BD, Schandler SL: Comparative analysis of paraspinal and frontalis EMG, heart rate and skin conductance in chronic low back pain patients and normals to various postures and stress. Scan J Rehab Med 14:39-46, 1982.
49. Ahern DK, Follick MJ, Council JR, Laser-Wolston N: Reliability of lumbar paravertebral EMG assessment in chronic low back pain. Arch Phys Med Rehabil 67:762-765, 1986.
50. Bernard TN: Don't discard diskography. (Letter) Radiology 162:285, 1987.
51. Errico TJ: The role of diskography in the 1980s. (Letter) Radiology 162:285-286, 1987.
52. Shapiro R: Current status of lumbar diskography (letter). Radiology 159:815, 1986.

53. Scullin DR: Lumbar diskography (letter). Radiology 162:284, 1987.
54. Weisel SW, Feffer HL, Rothman RH: Industrial low back pain: A comprehensive approach. Charlottesville, VA: Miche, 1985, 494.
55. Grubb SA, Lipscomb HJ, Guilford WB: The relative value of lumbar roentgenograms, metrizamide myelography, and discography in the assessment of patients with chronic low-back syndrome. Spine 12:282-285, 1987.
56. Kostuik JP: Decision-making in adult scoliosis. Spine 4:521-525, 1979.
57. Schutte HE, Park WM: The diagnostic value of bone scintigraphy in patients with low back pain. Skeletal Radiol 10:1-4, 1983.
58. Johansen JP, Fossgreen J, Hansen HH: Bone scanning in lumbar disc herniation. Acta Orthop Scand 51:617-620, 1980.
59. Schaffer DL, Pendergrass HP: Comparison of enzymes, radiographs and radionuclide methods of detecting bone metastases from carcinoma of the prostrate. Radiology 121:431, 1976.

CHAPTER 4

Treatment

Introduction

Most acute back pain is effectively treated with bedrest, analgesics, heat and time. There is rarely a need to hospitalize a patient with acute pain, even those with sciatica. If acute pain persists after a week (the period of time needed for return to work of 60% of all back cases), a course of primary conservative treatment is warranted for the next several weeks. Non-steroidal anti-inflammatory drugs, local heat application, and home exercise are commonly initiated at this juncture. Almost all patients with sciatica and without major or progressive neurological deficit should undergo this treatment without delay.

The literature indicates that approximately 90% of all patients with low back symptoms will return to work within six to twelve weeks of the onset of pain [1]. The unresponsive case requires a more aggressive form of conservative treatment that falls just short of surgery. The possible modalities include supervised exercise, traction, manipulation, massage, ultrasound, heat, ice, diathermy, eletrotherapy, biofeedback, inversion therapy, and back school. This second, more aggressive phase serves at least two purposes. Additional conservative treatment allows time for the body to heal itself. It also provides an opportunity to document the etiology of back pain in much greater detail. The physician can correlate radiographic evidence with findings from the physical examination, patient history, and the patient's response to various non-surgical treatments. In this way, the physician can develop a future strategy of more intensive management (e.g. surgical intervention) to be called into action if the back condition remains unresolved or deteriorates.

This chapter will discuss a wide variety of treatments, ranging from bedrest to percutaneous discectomy. In discussing the role each modality plays in the treatment of lumbar pathology, various techniques will be presented in a chronological sequence, structured according to the complexity and duration of pathology. The section will begin with the most common conservative remedies prescribed for the acute back problem (pain less than four weeks), such as bedrest and analgesics. The next phase of treatment remains conservative, but is expanded in scope to include a more intensive program designed to remedy persisting back pain which has not resolved within the initial four-week period. With lingering back pain, a more aggressive approach is necessary to prevent the relatively few case of unresolved back pain from becoming chronic patients (pain in excess of 8-12 weeks). Seventy-five percent of all back problems are rehabilitated within four weeks. For those subacute patients still requiring treatment, such modalities as EMG biofeedback, traction, acupuncture, epidural injection, and manipulation are but a few of the more complex techniques offered. After the more aggressive phase of conservative treatment has failed to relieve a patient's symptoms, additional strategies may be considered, including possible surgical intervention.

As an aid in the the critical review of treatment modalities, it would be helpful to clarify the therapeutic intentions underlying the techniques to be described. A list of some fundamental objectives encompassing the spectrum of current lumbar therapy was compiled by the editors of Spine [2]. The ten most relevant therapeutic objectives are as follows:

1. To promote rest for the affected anatomic structures, enhancing the natural mechanism of healing, while preventing aggravation of pain. Modalities include bedrest, spinal corsets and braces.
2. To diminish muscle spasm. Prevention of the development of a painspasm cycle with EMG biofeedback, manipulation and massage.
3. To diminish inflammation. Often the first step in treatment of a mechanical problem, modalities include systemic and local medication (epidural steriod injection, analgesics, oral steroids, other drugs).
4. To reduce pain, achieved by medication, acupuncture, electroacupuncture, TENS.
5. To increase strength (especially the torso muscles), with well supervised exercises and back school rehabilitation programs.
6. To increase the range of motion. Prevention of persistent spasm and prolonged inactivity by using traction and manipulation.
7. To increase endurance. Prevention of muscular atrophy with supervised exercise and back school programs.
8. To alter mechanical structures. Surgical modification achieved by discectomy, and fusion.
9. To alter neurologic structures. Denervation via rhizotomy.
10. To modify the psychosocial aspects of back pain. Particularly essential to treatment of the chronic case, as disability and illness behavior become increasingly disassociated from their original physical basis.

Finally, it is important that the reader understand the methodological problems that impede the design of adequate low back pain research data. The first problem is that back pain tends to improve spontaneously with time. It is difficult to establish the effectiveness of treatment in prospective randomized trials for a disease in which 9 out of 10 low back pain patients will improve within six to twelve weeks, regardless of the treatment modality. Secondly, partly because of problems in establishing diagnosis in patients with LBP, it is difficult to select homogeneous groups of patients on which to test the effect of a treatment. Controlled studies are few and far between. Rarely are sufficient patient characteristics provided, particularly the crucial distinction between acute, subacute and chronic cases. Moreover, conventional outcome measures, such as the presence of abnormal physical signs, or the ability of the patient to return to work, are very crude. Typically, only post-treatment measures are collected with no long-term follow-up. As a rule, a given treatment will appear much more successful when followed for only six months rather than over the course of ten or twenty years. In many studies, the sole criteria of the success or failure of a given treatment is left to the subjective impressions of the patient. A subject's lack of sensitivity may lead to failure in detecting a genuine treatment effect.

Consertive Treatment

Bedrest (Strict versus Light Activity)

Many authors feel an adequate period of bedrest is the most important element of therapy in the treatment of acute lumbar pain, especially disc related pain. The rationale behind bedrest is borne out by several observations. Since the natural history of low back pain is such that 80% to 90% of all acute back problems are resolved within 8 weeks regardless of treatment, there is little need for complicated treatment. Secondly, biomechanical research by Nachemson has calculated that intervertebral disc pressure can be dramatically reduced with horizontal posture [3]. If one assumes an association between increased disc pressure and increased severity of symptoms, it is logical that conservative management begin with bedrest.

Most doctors recommend that the patient should remain in bed with the exception of bathroom privileges. The patient should be placed in a position of pelvic tilt, reversing the lordotic curve and thereby stretching the ligaments, muscles and other soft-tissue that might be compressed or irritated. The ideal position is achieved when the hips and knees are flexed to a moderate, but comfortable degree, with the legs elevated on a chair or cushion. This posture is particularly important for acute disc herniation cases, as it allows a reduction of nerve root tension and inflammation by providing the maximum degree of foraminal space for the nerve to pass over or around the herniated disc material. The legitimacy of continuous pelvic tilt is explained by Rothman in this way: "Bedrest is important so that the secondary inflammatory reaction to disc degeneration may subside... If the edema and hyperemia of the soft tissues and nerve roots surrounding the extruded fragment are allowed to subside, the patient will become free of acute back pain and sciatica. This relief may or may not be permanent" [4].

Waddell counters this opinion with a well documented report, arguing that pain relief due to lying down was observed in only 58% of a 500 patient sample [5]. It is claimed that the only population group to which bedrest is of any benefit is the 1% to 2% of back cases with confirmed disc herniation or sciatica. In fact, very few controlled studies have shown a definite advantage of bedrest in the treatment of non-specific low-back pain. For example, Gilbert found no significant differences between bed rest, exercise and no treatment at all [6]. The same results were seen in a report by Lindstrom et al, the only difference between exercise and bed rest being an improvement in muscle strength with exercise[7]. Most research, however, agrees that the 1% to 2% of back cases with confirmed disc herniation can benefit from bedrest.

The number of days a patient should be confined to rest is highly variable, dependent upon the severity of the problem as perceived by the doctor and the extent to which the prescription is tolerated by the patient. On the basis of published research, reasonable bedrest recommendations may range from less than three days to two weeks. In an attempt to discover the answer to how much is enough for the acute back problem, Deyo et al. compared the consequences of prescribing two days of bed rest versus seven days of bed rest in a randomized trial of 203 patients [8]. Follow-up data was obtained at three weeks and three months after treatment. With the exception of one result, none of the outcome measures — functional status, perceptions, or symptoms – showed significant differences between the two groups. Those assigned to two days of bed rest missed substantially less work than those assigned to seven days (3.1 versus 5.6). The difference in the average number of days absent was 2.5, which represented a 45% reduction in the number of days lost. The fact that seven days of bedrest is no more efficacious than two days is highly relevant to the stratospheric levels of American worker absenteeism in a country that missed 1400 days per 1000 workers as a result of back pain, especially when one recognizes that bedrest is by far the most commonly prescribed treatment.

Deyo is quick to point out that two day treatment is only suitable for those low back patients with injuries of the muscles, ligaments and facet joints. Individuals with disc herniation and neurologic deficits are very likely to require more prolonged bedrest. One should also note that since the study was conducted in a primary care setting, the nature and severity of back problems may differ substantially from those seen in a specialty practice, like orthopedics. It is suggested that the two day treatment strategy might not be suitable in an environment of potentially more complex cases of lumbar pathology. Finally, cultural factors may have influenced the results of the study, as the great majority of the participants were Hispanic. The ability to tolerate pain is thought by many to be influenced by the racial and socioeconomic environment of the patient. Therefore a generalization of the results should be carefully qualified.

Other studies have confirmed the validity of bedrest. Weisel et al, evaluated the efficacy of bedrest in 80 combat recruits having back pain with no signs of neural tension or sciatica [9]. The study had soldiers randomly assigned to groups receiving continuous bed rest or ambulation (but excused from physical activity). Results indicated thaт the average interval for return to full activity was 50% less for those treated by bedrest than by ambulation (6.6 days versus 11.5 days). The bedrest group also experienced 60% less pain. Waddell argues that several methodological considerations cast doubt on the conclusiveness of Weisel's report. Apparently, no allowance was made for the patient's attitudes to the treatment or to training, while observer bias in assessing results should not be dismissed as irrelevant.

Exercise

As the preceding reports indicate, the very heart of the controversy is a "rest versus recovery debate," which implies passive versus active rehabilitation. Waddell clearly supports the aggressive rehabilitation of the patient, conscious not only of the paucity of favorable scientific evidence supporting bed rest, but also concerned with the deleterious side-effects of prolonged bed rest, such as bone demineralization, a 3% loss of muscle strength per day, decreased physical fitness, and possibly an inhibited healing process due to muscular stiffness. Joint tightness and contracture can also occur, restricting the normal range of motion. There is a high probability of decreased vital capacity in the respiratory system, decreased maximal ventilation, and reduced ability to cough. Should the decision be made to operate, the deconditioned patient goes into surgery at a distinct disadvantage. As Nutter states, the patient is "more likely to suffer from medical complications such as pneumonia or deep vein thrombosis following surgery. Any complication requires extra bedrest, delays rehabilitation, and causes further deterioration from immobility" [10].

On the other hand, there is evidence that increased activity may promote bone and muscle strength, improve disc and cartilage nutrition (a core belief of Nachemson), improve posture, stabilize hypermobile segments and perhaps most importantly, stimulate endorphin levels to reduce the sensitivity to pain [11]. It has been suggested that people who exercise sufficiently are able to increase levels of beta-endorphins in their blood and spinal fluid, allowing patients with back pain to feel better during and after exercise. Some investigators have actually suggested that exercise can reverse the direction of nucleus pulposus bulging and reduce nerve root compression. As opposed to strict bedrest, it is argued that the most effective conservative treatment is bedrest for short periods, interspersed with light activity to avoid muscular atrophy and stiffness. Bigos recommends that the patient take three or four walks per day to combat the debilitating effects of bed rest, including muscular deconditioning [12].

In addition to physical benefits, exercise also has a positive psychological influence which is essential in preventing a relatively benign acute injury from becoming a debilitating chronic condition. All too often, patients rely on such passive conservative treatments as manipulation, medication, massage, ultrasound, TENS, and biofeedback to cure their back pain. Unfortunately, there is no magical panacea that guarantees a cure while the patient seems as much a spectator to treatment as the doctor. As an alternative to passive treatment, exercise requires the active participation of the patient. Unlike other modalities, exercise instills confidence in the patient that he does not have a serious back disease and that movement will not cause further deterioration. As the reader will discover in the chronic pain chapter, this sense of confidence is often crucial to recovery. If the patient allows himself to decrease function solely because of pain and not because of any true risk of further injury, the development of illness behavior and chronic disability may result.

Even in the case of acute disc herniation, the stress of walking or partaking in mild daily activities does not appear to increase the risk of worsening the condition [13]. In fact, activities such as speed walking, cycling, swimming, even jogging or jumping up and down have not been found to produce intradiscal pressures as high as sitting, which can be nearly twice as much as standing pressure. In the absence of bone or joint instability, Bigos argues that such excercise be incorporated into rehabilitation as soon as possible. While it might appear premature to expose a tender back problem to potentially vigorous activity, some research has indicated that pain can actually be diminished with exercise. Several investigations have demonstrated that patients with low-back pain or sciatica can do selected activities almost normally, without increasing their pain. Fordyce, for instance, reports that subjective complaints of pain are largely unrelated to actual activity levels, and that observed pain behavior is actually inversely proportional to the amount of exercise done [14]. Lewis has indicated that aerobic exercises increase the body's production of beta-endorphins, which are thought to play an important role in diminishing pain perception [15]. Considering these findings detailing the merits of exercise, Waddell writes: "There is strongly suggestive evidence that rest, particularly prolonged bed rest, may be the most harmful treatment ever devised and a potent cause of iatrogenic disability."

Medication

Drug therapy for low back pain can be divided into four distinct categories: steroidal and non-steroidal anti-inflammatories, analgesics, muscle relaxants, and anti-depressants.

The underlying logic of anti-inflammatory treatment is based on the mechanics of the inflammatory response that is thought to trigger pain, usually caused by neural compression (i.e. root entrapment syndrome). These medications block prostaglandin production and thereby reduce inflammation, which in turn promotes healing and reduces pain. The research on anti-inflammatory agents is equivocal, many of the studies failing to quantify the contributing effects of bedrest prescribed along with the various medications. Ibuprofen (Motrin), sulindac (Clinoril), phenylbutazone (Butazolidin), and oxyphenylbutazone (Tandearil) have all been reported successful in back treatment. Cortisone is a very potent steroidal anti-inflammatory, and should not be used excessively. Cortisone is most effective when injected over the facet joint or the inflammed nerve root of patients with demonstrated nerve root irritation. Selby recommends non-steroidal anti-inflammatory drugs as the "single most useful medication in non-specific low back pain" [16]. Although these drugs have fewer complications than their steroidal counterparts, they may also be much less effective.

Aspirin appears to be the most commonly prescribed analgesic (also considered a non-steroidal anti-inflammatory) endorsed in conjunction with bedrest by the leading back scholars, including Nachemson, Rothman and Frymoyer [17-19]. There are no known non-addicting analgesics that are much better than aspirin. In those cases where aspirin is not well tolerated (usually due to gastrointestinal intolerance), acetaminophen (e g Tylenol) is commonly substituted. Aspirin, acetaminophen with codeine (e g Tylenol #3), oxycodone with aspirin (e g Percodan), naproxen (Naprosyn), and diflunisal (Dolobid) are all effective analgesics, according to Frymoyer [19]. If additional pain relief is required, narcotic analgesics such as codeine, oxycodone, or propoxyphene (e.g. Darvon) can be prescribed. Caution must be exercised during the administration of these narcotics, as they are addictive, and can be lethal when combined with alcohol. Rothman writes: "Although analgesics undoubtedly relieve pain for brief periods, tolerance, habit formation and side-effects pose various problems and make their prolonged use not advisable" [4].

Muscle relaxants are used with the assumption that pain is coming from the muscle spasm. Yet the most commonly used relaxants have little peripheral effect on spasm. Benzodiazepine derivatives are commonly prescribed, including diazepam (e g Valium), clorazepate (Tronxene), and oxazepam (Serax). The principal benefits of these drugs seems to be their strong sedative capabilities. Consequently, they are addictive; abrupt withdrawal may cause extreme agitation, sleeplessness, and even convulsions. It has not been proven that muscle relaxants make a significant difference in the clinical course of low back pain.

Anti-depressants are used in the treatment of depression which often accompanies chronic low back pain. The tricyclic anti-depressants have been found to be the most useful group of drugs for such patients. Reversal of depression and pain reduction can result. Carron recommends amitriptyline (e g Elavil) for those patients with sleep disturbances and agitation, and imipramine (e g

Tofronil) for patients with decreased psychomotor activity [20]. Doxepin (e g Sinequan) is suggested as the drug of choice in patients with masked depression and associated anxiety. Gingras found imipramine superior to placebo in patients with arthritic pain [21]. Among the most troublesome side-effects of these tricyclic drugs are dryness of the mouth, constipation, and urinary retention.

In conclusion, White is not alone in his assessment of the pharmacological treatment of back pain when he remarks: "Medication is probably the least valuable tool in the treatment of low back pain. Medication does not change the underlying condition, nor does it change the abusive factors that have led to the condition. It "covers up" the symptoms rather than encouraging the patient to accept responsibility for the symptoms. With the symptoms covered up, the underlying condition continues on unabated and becomes a severe condition" [22].

Traction

Traction is a time-honored conservative procedure which has been used in the management of low back pathology for the past several centuries. Traction can be applied by means of autotraction, gravity reduction, and motorized techniques. The most popular type of traction is pelvic traction, which employs a snug canvas girdle encircling the pelvis and hips and attached to weights hung at the foot of the bed. The fundamental principle involved in its utilization is an unloading of the spine by stretching muscles and ligaments, eventually reducing intradiscal pressure. Theoretically, the increased mechanical effects of leverage will distract the posterior elements of the vertebral column, reversing the lumbar lordosis of the spine, reducing compression upon the posterior portion of the annulus fibrosis, and increasing the aperture of the intervertebral foramina. Unfortunately, the realization of this objective is more apparent than real. Research indicates that a distraction force equivalent to 60% of body weight will reduce intradiscal pressure at L3 only 25% when the patient is standing [23]. Even in a horizontal position, an intradiscal pressure reduction of only 20% to 30% is realized when as much as 30 kilos of traction are applied for three seconds.

The value of traction beyond a placebo affect has not been demonstrated, particularly in controlled studies. Most believe that the positive results of traction are not due to mechanical benefits, but rather to keeping the patient in bed. Rothman has found that traction is occasionally helpful in enforcing a prescription of bedrest, which some feel is the most important facet of conservative management. Finneson comments that traction may do no more than "alleviate the monotony of bed rest and be of psychological advantage in imparting to the patient a sense of active therapy" [24]. An assessment of efficacy is further complicated by parameters such as preparation of the patient, posture, friction, traction angle, intensity and type of apparatus. Claims that disk herniations can be reduced have not been proven.

A double-blind study by Weber of the effects of traction on sciatic patients found no significant statistical differences in relief of symptoms between the groups receiving real and simulated traction [25]. The same study also reported that traction had no effect on spinal mobility, tension signs, deep tendon reflexes, paresis, sensory deficit, or the consumption of analgesics. However, Weber did acknowledge a positive psychologic effect from the patient's expectations for recovery while in traction. Christie reported similar results in an early single-blind trial of treatment with traction compared with an analgesic [26]. Assessment after a four week period showed no overall differences. A more recent single-blind study of 72 patients treated with intermittent traction of 20 minutes duration for 5 to 7 days showed no evidence of efficacy [26]. Pal et al. conducted a controlled, double-blind trial on 41 patients, randomly selected to receive either continuous lumbar traction of 5.5 to 8.2 kg or continuous traction of only 1.4 to 1.8 kg [27]. While the consumption of analgesics was significantly reduced by both groups within a two week period, at no time was there any statistically significant difference in analgesic consumption, pain score, or straight-leg angle between the two groups. Pal remarks: "The results of our trial indicate that conventional continuous traction carries no advantage over simulated traction. This would support the view that any benefit from continuous traction derives from the enforced immobilization.... It may be that minimal-weight traction at home as a complement to complete bed rest may have an important place and might obviate the need for costly hospitalization."

Equivocal results were also reported by Mathews et al. [28]. A total of 143 patients with lumbar nerve root pain, dural tension signs, limited back movement and back pain were randomly assigned to a group receiving traction and a control group receiving infra-red heat treatment. A comparison of the two-week treatment program revealed that 40/77 (52%) of those treated with traction and 27/54 (50%) of the control group had recovered in the period. Although the traction nearly always relieved pain while the patient was in treatment, relief was only temporary. Although a higher proportion of treated patients were improved on the 7th day, with the difference expanded until the end of the two weeks, specific differences between the two groups achieved only borderline significance.

Spinal Orthoses – Braces and Corsets

As an aid in the splinting of the spine, corsets and braces are among the least expensive and most widely used treatment remedies. A brace is a compromise between bedrest and function. While there is no concrete scientific evidence of clinical effectiveness, retrospective studies have reported a 30% to 80% improvement of symptoms. Frymoyer, for instance, endorses the use of spinal bracing in patients with osteoporotic compression fractures, spondylolisthesis, "segmental instability," and in some patients with spinal stenosis [19]. Several theories have been proposed that explain how corsets can reduce back pain. One of the most publicized theories concerns the role of intrabdominal pressure. It is thought that the corset acts as an abdominal binder, thus raising the abdominal pressure and redistributing a portion of the load from the spine to the abdominal muscles and diaphragm. Morris found that lumbar braces increased the intra-abdominal pressure of the wearer at rest by compressing the abdomen [29]. Much like the wide support belts that enable weight lifters to lift extraordinarily heavy weights by generating artificially high hydraulic forces, a tight corset is believed to act in the same way, by limiting the stress on the spine and thus the symptoms of back pain [30].

Restriction of motion is another primary mechanical function of the corset and brace, preventing the patient from undertaking movement that might precipitate pain. A corset that limits upper body flexion, extension or lateral bending will tend to keep lumbar trunk loads small. Mobility reduction is most effectively accomplished by a brace. However, because of the wide variability of lumbar corset designs, there is much uncertainty regarding the amount of back movement restriction. Various studies have explored the extent of actual restricted motion by evaluating the most common mechanical criteria related to potential back pain, including gross spine motion [31], intersegmental motion [32,33], myoelectric activity of trunk muscles [34], intra-abdominal pressure [35], and intradiscal pressure [36]. What follows is a cross-section of current research describing the inconsistent efficacy rates of corsets or braces as measured by the mechanical variables just listed [31-36]. Paradoxically, it will be shown that some of these studies are able to demonstrate varying degrees of pain reduction, despite scientific measurement documenting an inability to restrict motion or reduce muscle activity in any consistent manner.

In a report dealing exclusively with the biomechanical aspects of corset use, Nachemson et al. evaluated intradiscal pressures, intra-gastric pressures and myolelectric trunk muscle activities in four volunteers wearing five different braces or corsets while performing six tasks [37]. All of the participants were in good health, with no history of back injury or significant back pain. The subjects were asked to perform the tasks while standing, with and without braces. The orthoses studied were a Camp canvas corset, a Raney flexion jacket, and three kinds of Boston braces.

Results of the trial showed a significant degree of ambiguity. Intradiscal pressure was found to be lower in two-thirds of the excercises, and higher in one-third, when compared to the no-orthoses data. Intra-abdominal pressure developed over the exercises were generally low, with no clear trends indicating what effect the wearing of a brace/corset had on the measurements. This can be compared to the observations of Morris, who found a decrease in myolelectric activities of the abdominal muscles when braces were worn [35]. The same inconsistent finding was seen in the myoelectric data of the erector spinae, and abdominal muscles. Nachemson notes that erector spinae muscle activity decreased when a brace/corset was worn in fewer than half of the tasks studied, while abdominal muscle activity decreased when an orthosis was worn in over 75% of the cases studied. A limited endorsement of corsets and braces is put forth: "Our findings suggest that the wearing of an orthosis can at least sometimes result in significant unloading of lumbar trunk structures... No one orthosis we examined seemed clearly superior to another in mechanical effectiveness in the tasks studied here" [37].

The above statement can be contrasted with Schroeder's remarks: "A back support can restrict, but not prevent motion in the lower lumbar region. It seems highly unlikely that any device applied to the body can effectively splint the lumbosacral region" [38]. Quinet et al. goes even further in a complete condemnation of corset and braces: "The widespread use of these gimmicks ought to be curtailed until we have data suggesting that our patients are more likely to profit from their continued use than are orthopedic supply homes" [39].

Grew et al. confirmed that spinal supports influenced the postural mechanics, intra-abdominal pressure and skin temperature of a group of male low back pain patients given corsets [40]. As with the Nachemson study, five types of orthoses were evaluated; very few differences were noted. The most important distinction between supports was considerable variation in the reduction of spinal mobility. A rigid form of bracing was found to be essential to significant mobility reduction. Corsets made of fabric and elastic provided little restriction of movement. All the spinal supports raised the resting level of intra-abdominal pressure in all postures, with no differences noted between supports. However, braces and corsets had no effect during excercise.

Reference was made to the dangers of long-term support treatment, emphasizing the subconscious adoption of the orthosis as part of the patient's support mechanism. Grew points out that a reduction in abdominal muscle acitivity in those patients using corsets was probably responsible for the fact that only one patient had a resting intra-abdominal pressure comparable with the untreated group. It is generally recognized that prolonged reliance will reduce the need for activation of the abdominal musculature while a psychologic and physiologic dependence is created, leading to atrophy and the potential for additional injury. It can be expected that at some point, the use of a spinal support can result in a vicious circle, where the intra-abdominal pressure the treatment was meant to stabilize and strengthen is continuously eroded the longer the support is utilized. Thus, Grew recommends that after two to three weeks, orthosis be discontinued.

Million randomly allocated a group of 19 chronic low back patients to corset treatment with and without a plastic insert spinal support [30]. A global subjective index found a highly significant improvement in the patients with the spinal support, but minimal change in those treated without the insert.

Specifically, improvement was noted with respect to pain at night and in bed, interference with life-style and work, and discomfort when walking. Improvement for the placebo group was only noted by a reduction of pain when lying down. However, the global index improved for all patients over the study period. An objective assessment was also conducted. Improvement in extension and flexion was seen in the spinal support group, while improvement in straight-leg-raising and extension was observed among the placebo group. It was also found that the objective index for all patients showed improvement over the study period but with no differences between groups.

Transcutaneous Electrical Nerve Stimulation (TENS)

TENS is a technique aimed at reducing the physiologic perception of pain through the use of an electrical stimulator. Electrodes are applied to the area of pain, generally the site of a myofascial "trigger point". The basis for the development of TENS lies in the early work of Melzack and Wall, who theorized that repetitive stimulation of cutaneous afferent nerves would "gate" or block back pain by serving as a counter-irritant [41]. The "gate-control" model postulates that stimulation might activate descending inhibitory mechanisms or might compete at the spinal level with ascending noxious input. Furthermore, more current theory has speculated upon the role that endogenous natural opiates might play in pain reduction via electrical stimulation.

Although the management of lumbar pain by the use of TENS is well documented in the literature, its effectiveness is heavily disputed. An uncontrolled TENS trial by Fried et al. in a group of 846 patients with chronic pain (72% of them back-related) showed improvement in 84% of the respondents [42]. Most of the injuries were the result of industrial trauma, sustained on average 5 months before admission to the study. Among those who returned to work, 86.4% claimed continued benefit from TENS, compared to 82% for the subgroup not working. This high rate of pain relief must be considered with caution, as each patient also received a full range of therapy appropriate to their disability, which almost certainly contributed to the efficacy of TENS treatment.

According to Procacci et al, patients were most likely to benefit from TENS if trigger points were present [43]. Based upon the results of 108 patients, it was found that pain disappeared or diminished in all cases. The period of pain relief was dependent upon the nature of two key pathophysiological mechanisms. Those patients with typical trigger points showed the longest period of pain relief, in excess of two months in some cases. Only temporary relief of 2 to 3 hours was observed in those patients presenting signs of denervation and lacking trigger points. The effects of afferent stimulation on the nervous system are less effective when peripheral afferent fibers have been damaged, blood vessels are severed, and severe circulatory disturbance persists.

Indeck and Printy tested 35 patients, finding 23 to have 50% to 89% pain relief, while the remainder claimed complete pain relief [44]. An average pain relief rate of 60% was reported by Melzack in his use of brief, intense TENS at trigger points [45]. The duration of pain relief was found to vary from hours to days. A comparison between TENS and acupuncture by Fox and Melzack revealed that pain relief was greater than 33% in 75% of the patients receiving acupuncture and in 66% of the patients receiving TENS [46]. Another comparative evaluation by Melzack treated 44 chronic low back patients with TENS and ice massage, yielding a 33% reduction of pain in 67% of the patients (as demonstrated on the McGill Pain Questionnaire) [47]. While the average length of pain relief was 10 hours, both treatments were equally effective. Continued pain relief was not demonstrated. It was concluded that the treatment did not accelerate return to work or to a normal degree of functioning.

Other segments of the literature have found dead-battery TENS treatment to be nearly as effective as the real thing. Thoresteinsson et al. compared TENS with a placebo (TENS electrode attachments with no current) in a sample study of 93 chronic pain patients [48]. Included in the group were 38 chronic back patients. Immediately following treatment, the patients reported complete or partial pain relief in 48% of the TENS trials and in 32% of the placebo trials. Long term pain relief at 3 and 6 months rapidly diminished. It should be noted that the placebo effects in this study were uncontrolled. Lehmann et al. assigned 54 patients to three treatment groups: TENS, dead-battery TENS, and electroacupuncture [49]. All of the participants had low back pain for greater than six months. Based upon results from the Visual Analog Scale and disability assessment by both physician and patient, there were no differences between treatment groups with respect to their overall rehabilitation. In fact, all three groups ranked the contribution of education as being greater than electrical stimulation of any kind.

Acupuncture and Electroacupuncture

Acupuncture is a therapy characterized by the insertion of needles at predetermined sites in cutaneous and subcutaneous tissues. There are no scientific studies demonstrating the superiority of acupuncture over other treatment modalities, although a few studies have reported a reduction in chronic back pain. Electroacupuncture is closely related to TENS, and is useful in a number of conditions other than musculoskeletal pain, especially in the treatment of soft-tissue injuries. In a study by Santiesteban, ten subjects randomly assigned to an eletroacupuncture group or a physical therapy group indicated that electroacupuncture significantly relieved pain and increased range of motion when compared to traditional physical therapy [50].

A double-blind, placebo-controlled trial of 77 patients completely contradicts the preceding observations, finding placebo and acupuncture to be equally efficacious in an 18 week evaluation by Mendelson et al.[51]. A realistic placebo was achieved by placing needles at non-acupuncture, non-tender sites previously infiltrated with a small volume of local anesthetic and inserting the needles superficially without stimulation. In the first four-week phase of the trial, acupuncture led to satisfactory pain relief in 40% of those patients, versus 26% for placebo. The second four-week period showed the placebo group reporting 40% pain reduction, compared with 19% for the acupuncture group. The difference between the two groups was significant only in the second phase of the trial, with placebo treatment considered more effective. Overall, no difference in the effectiveness of acupuncture and placebo was observed. Other studies confirming acupuncture to be no better than placebo include separate reports by Lee, Gaw, and Moore [52-54]. Similar findings by Edelist were shown in a trial of 30 patients suffering from painful disc disease [55]. Unable to respond to conventional treatment, the patients were randomly divided into a group receiving acupuncture and another group given sham acupunture treatment. After three treatments, there was no difference in response between the two groups in either subjective or objective pain reduction.

MacDonald et al. conducted a considerably smaller single-blind, placebo-controlled, randomized study comparing 8 patients treated by acupuncture and 9 patients treated by placebo [56]. Administration of placebo was characterized by the insertion of needles superficially into the skin and subcutaneous layers to a depth of 4 mm for short periods of time once a week. Each patient had at least a one year history of back pain. In all five measures of efficacy chosen for the study (pain scores, activity pain scores, physical signs, severity, and area of pain), the acupunture group attained higher pain relief than the control group. Furthermore, it was concluded that it is not necessary to enter the muscle itself to achieve a significant benefit when compared to the effects placebo.

Low Back Schools

Low back schools were developed nearly twenty years ago in Sweden. Although there are considerable differences in the curriculum, nearly all programs include educational material concerning the anatomy and physiology of the back, rest positions, proper body mechanics and work techniques. Additionally, the more comprehensive back school regimens emphasize a work hardening program based upon careful analysis of the worker's job tasks, a suitable excercise program structured to the patient's specific needs, and relaxation training for stress and pain management. In short, all low back schools draw upon particular aspects of physical, psychological and occupational therapy that are consistent with the overall objectives of the program.

Treatment goals include increasing the patient's self-care, prevention of recurrences, muscle strengthening (especially through back flexion and extension exercises), and application of musculoskeletal education to the work place (ergonomics). The total number of sessions can range from two to forty. According to an exhaustive 1987 review of low back schools, Linton states that most of the programs provide an average of four hours of instruction in four separate sessions [57]. Typically, back schools have been oriented toward patients with chronic or recurrent problems, although the current trend seems to be an increased emphasis on back pain prevention in acute cases.

Studies on the efficacy of treatment are most easily organized into controlled and uncontrolled evaluations. Not surprisingly, most uncontrolled studies demonstrate overwhelmingly positive evidence which must be interpreted with substantial caution. For instance, a report by Hall et al. presents results based upon a follow-up questionnaire return rate of only 38% [58]. A more critical uncontrolled trial by Kvien et al. compared a low back school group with a group receiving traditional physical therapy, hydroptherapy and electrical stimulation [59]. The results of a one-year follow-up found no significant differences in subjective pain ratings, daily activities, recreational walking, or employment, although fewer patients in the back school group reported having received physical therapy during the period.

More conclusive evidence is observed in controlled studies. Bergquist-Ullman et al. assigned 217 auto workers with acute or subacute low back pain to one of three groups: back school, combined physical therapy, and placebo treatment [60]. Those workers in the back school group had a significantly shorter duration of symptoms than the controlled group, and the same duration as the physical therapy group. Significantly, workers in the back school group had the shortest duration of sick leave during the initial pain episode, yet no significant differences between the groups were observed on the pain index. A year after completion of treatment, no differences were found between any of the groups with regard to the incidence or duration of recurrences or number of sick days. It was concluded that back school and therapy were more efficacious than placebo.

Two groups of nursing aides suffering from acute low back pain were selected by Dehlin for physical fitness training or ergonomic counseling, and compared with a control group receiving simulated instruction [61]. No significant difference was seen between the groups for self-rated psychological perception of work, except for the variable of coworker relations, where the physical fitness group performed better. In terms of low back symptoms pain intensity and frequency, use of analgesiscs, and work capacity, similar improvement patterns were observed in both groups, with no significant differences.

Similar findings by Lindequist and Gilbert also argue against the notion of back school as a better alternative to low back pain management [62-63]. Lindequist was unable to report any differences between a group given detailed, individualized information emphasizing back strain prevention, and a control group offered simple advice and analgesics. Back school and physical therapy were considered to be more harmful than beneficial by Gilbert, in an evaluation of back school versus bedrest or no treatment at all. No significant differences between back school and control treatment were found by Ljungberg in an evaluation of 5000 government employees with back or neck pain [64]. Another report unable to document the efficacy of back school was conducted by Aberg, who compared subjects in a six-week inpatient treatment program consisting of physical therapy, low back school and vocational training [65]. Those on the waiting list for the program served as the control group. No significant changes were observed regarding employment status, number of sick days, pain, health, social activities or work capacity, although the treated group had a more optimistic perspective than the controls about training the back and preventing further back injury. This psychological component should not be easily dismissed, as it is noted by several reporters as one of the most significant aspects of treatment, playing a crucial role in successful rehabilitation.

While nearly all of the preceding studies admitted only subjects with acute back pain, Lankhorst evaluated the merits of back school on a population of chronic low back patients [66]. A Swedish back school group was compared to a group receiving placebo treatment. With regard to pain, function, spinal mobility and other standardized measures, no significant positive effects for either group was noted. One year after treatment, the same findings remained intact. It was ultimately concluded that low back school was of minimal value in the chronic phase of low back pain. Slightly more favorable results were submitted by Moffett et al. in a comparative evaluation of groups receiving low back school or abdominal excercise [67]. While both groups tended to improve, those in the low back school increased their activity levels more than the excercise group. After a one-year follow-up, negligible differences were observed in either group, which correlates with the general belief that the positive effects of low back school inevitably disappear almost completely within one year in chronic low back patients.

The results of a two-year study of an aggressive back school approach to functional rehabilitation of chronic industrial low back injury documents very persuasive results supporting the efficacy of multidisciplinary treatment. Mayer et al. admitted 116 consecutive patients to a treatment program consisting of specific excercises, training in functional tasks, education, and work simulation/hardening [68]. Psychological training was an integral part of the program, emphasizing behavioral stress management, cognitive-behavioral skills, individual and group counseling, and family counseling. Results of this curriculum were compared to a control group of 72 untreated patients. At the one-year follow-up, 85% of the treatment group was either working or in a training program, contrasted to an employment rate of 39% for the control group and 13% for treatment dropouts. Distinct differences were observed in the number of additional surgeries: 50% of the treatment drop-out group, 20% of the controls, and only 9% of the treatment group underwent additional back surgery. Similar results were seen with respect to the percentage of patients visiting health care professionals: 75% of the controls, 67% of the treatment dropouts and 33% of the treatment group. There was an average of 16 visits made by the control group, 6.7 visits made by treatment dropouts, and only 3.6 visits made by the treatment group.

Mayer attributes the successful recovery of so many treated participants to the belief that return to work is not merely dependent upon an improvement in physical capacity, but is also fundamentally based upon a renewal of psychological motivation to become productive. According to the author, most back schools and pain clinics all too often ignore the psychological component of backache. The result is a tendency to treat the experience of pain, and not the disability associated with pain behavior.

Manipulation (Chiropractic)

Spinal joint manipulation is a procedure where the hands are used to mobilize, adjust, stimulate or otherwise influence the spinal and paraspinal tissues with the aim of influencing the patient's health. Manipulative therapy can be more specifically classified as manipulation, mobilization, manual traction, soft-tissue massage, or point-pressure technique. Dating back to the time of Hippocrates, manipulation is based on the assumption that "subluxation" of the vertabrae precipitates low back pain, and that these complaints can be reduced with correction of the "misalignment", (also referred to as an osteopathic lesion, vertebral fixation or blockage, or area of spinal or somatic dysfunction). Diagnosis of subluxation is based upon manual palpation of vertebral malposition, abnormal vertebral motion, abnormal joint play and end feel, and soft tissue abnormalities [69]. Manipulation is one of the most widely used methods of treating spinal pain. An estimated 90 million patients visited chiropractors in the United States in 1976, which increased to 120 million in 1980 [70]. At least 50% of these visits were related to low back pain. Osteopaths are also visited, though in smaller numbers

Mechanical, neurophysiologic and psychologic therapeutic benefits are said to result from manipulation. Mechanical therapy attacks the consequences of an immobilized joint, a condition where the connective tissues of the ligaments, muscles and fascia have lost their flexibility. It is speculated that manipulation causes a rupture of attached tissue fibers and any intra-articular capsular adhesions that may have formed, relieving muscle spasm and restoring freer motion. While most research demonstrates that the mechanical component of manipulation stops well short of reversing the course of lumbar disc herniation, a few authors have suggested that the prolapsed nucleus pulposus can be maneuvered by exertion of a centripetal pressure on the herniated material. The neurologic component of manipulation works in a manner similar to TENS or acupuncture, relieving pain by an inhibitory effect on afferent painful stimuli (via the "gate control" mechanism proposed by Melzack). Lastly, the psychological benefits of the "laying on of hands" is widely acknowledged by the medical community, enhancing the patient's perception of the interest, concern, and skills of the clinician. While there seems to be no lack of theory explaining the efficacy of this modality, the question of how manipulation relieves pain remains unanswered. For the time being, the efficacy of spinal manipulation is neither scientifically proven or disproven.

The clinical evaluation of manipulation has progressed slowly. Prior to 1975, no serious attempt to produce a blinded controlled trial was undertaken. To date, the literature still suffers from several important methodological shortcomings that make it exceedingly difficult to draw conclusions. A double-blind trial has proven impossible to structure with the modality because the treating clinician must be aware of the therapy employed. Such studies are further complicated by the fact that there is no generally accepted method to measure the disorders associated with low back pain. Additionally, nearly all studies that have demonstrated therapeutic value suffer from lack of adequate control for placebo effects. Many of the trials have used diathermy or analgesics to treat the control group, yet this is inadequate for a therapeutic modality such as manipulation because the effect from "laying on of the hands" may have a substantially more powerful placebo effect than an unplugged diathermy machine or saline solution.

There is a general consensus that manipulation is only beneficial in the short run, immediately following treatment and lasting no longer than two or three weeks. Effectiveness after three to twelve months is minimal. More specifically, the treatment is most beneficial in patients who have acute pain and no leg pain or neurologic deficits. Glover, for instance, found that only patients with acute low back pain responded with significant decrease in pain following a single rotary manipulation[71]. A more recent example is a single-blind, randomized controlled trial of rotational manipulation in 81 adults reported by Godfrey et al.[72]. Patients having acute lumbar pain of less than 14 days duration were distributed between the control group receiving minimal massage and low-level electrical stimulation and the treatment group. The criteria for efficacy included symptoms, daily activities, mobility and tenderness to palpation. Both groups showed a highly significant improvement during the 2 to 3 week observation period, yet at the end of treatment there was no statistically significant differences between the two groups on any the measurement criteria. The authors remark: "It may well be that manipulation is of some benefit in the recovery pattern of selected cases of acute low back pain, but the target group may be small and relatively inaccessible to the few physicians who are trained in manipulation."

Tobis et al. structured a trial with a possible alternative to the placebo problem described at the beginning of the section [73]. Patients without prior experience of manipulation were selected for a control group which only received soft tissue massage. Results were based upon a questionnaire regarding pain relief and any increased ability to perform simple tasks (dressing, walking, reaching, bending, etc..) immediately after the first treatment. In every category, those receiving actual manipulative therapy demonstrated greater improvement, yet by the time of discharge from the clinic, there was no difference between the two groups. According to Tobis, "manipulation appears to be effective primarily in accelerating recovery from an episode of back pain."

Nwuga compared the efficacy of manipulation to conventional back pain management (heat, pelvic tilt excercise, postural education, and lifting instructions) [77]. The 51 patients were all females with low back pain resulting from lumbar intervertebral disc herniation. Those patients treated with manipulation showed greater statistically significant improvement in total flexion and extension, total side flexion, total rotation, and straight-leg-raising values. Yet Doran et al. observed no differences between manipulation, physiotherapy, corset or analgesic treatment in 456 patients during follow-up examinations at three weeks, three months, and three years [75]. Another study by Sim-Williams et al. revealed that after three months, manipulation was no more effective than placebo in the treatment of a group of out-patients [76]. Hoelher reported the same tendency: at a 2-3 month follow-up, pain reduction among patients receiving manipulation and sham manipulation were 88% and 86%, respectively [77].

Manipulation was determined by Farrell to be more efficacious than conservative treatment in an evaluation of 48 subjects with acute low back pain and no neurologic signs [78]. Subjects were randomly assigned to either manipulation or a regimen of diathermy, isometric abdominal excercises and ergonomic instruction. Each subject was treated three times a week for up to three weeks. The findings indicated that patients treated with manipulation had a shorter mean duration of symptoms, and achieved symptom-free status with fewer sessions than the conservatively treated group. Moreover, these patients demonstrated a larger range of lumbar extension movements on the final day of treatment compared to the conservative group. Despite this tendency, no significant differences in subjective pain rating were noted between the two treatment groups at the end of three weeks.

Spinal manipulation is not without its adverse side effects. Common short-term reactions include autonomic disturbances such as faintness, perspiration, and overbreathing. Low back injury following manipulation is extremely rare because of the relatively great strength of the lumbar vertebral structures and the muscle mass surrounding them. However, there are certain spinal conditions that could be vulnerable to forceful manipulation such as patients with hypermobility, bone disease, and spinal lesions with neurological deficits. Lumbar disc herniation can be made worse by excessively forceful manipulation, possibly resulting in cauda equina syndrome.

Epidural Steroid Injection

The action mechanism of epidural injection, primarily steroids, has been debated extensively in the literature. Rather than a correction of the herniated disc, spondylosis, spinal stenosis, acute lumbar strain or other primary back problems, the goal of steroid injection is exclusively focused on the reduction of neural inflammation secondary to the structural pathology. Often times, the neural response to irritation caused by compression is the buildup of peridural, fibrotic adhesions which can cluster and cause the nerve to swell. Epidural injection is one method of reducing the buildup of peridural fibers by reducing swelling, inflammation and pain. It is thought that steroids operate in either a pharmacologic mode, or by altering the volume at the injected nerve site. The benefit of injecting the epidural space, the site at which the nerve roots pass before entering the intervertebral foramen, is that a concentrated amount of medication can be deposited and retained in a specific area, exposing the nerves to the medication for a prolonged period of time. While injection may be effective when nerve root irritation symptoms are present, it is not effective against non-specific low back pain. The most common side effect of injection is headache, resulting from pressure changes in the epidural space or inadvertent puncture of the arachnoid membrane. Aseptic meningitis, infection and increased neurological problems have also been reported.

The efficacy of epidural steroid injection has been periodically validated since 1953, when Lievre and associates were the first to utilize steroids epidurally in an attempt to relieve backpain. In 1957, Cappio reported successful pain relief in 67% of cases reviewed [79]. In 1961, Coomes compared epidural injection with bedrest in a prospective trial of 40 patients, demonstrating a more rapid recovery from pain in the injected group [80]. In another study, Dilke compared epidural injection of methylprednisolone to normal saline solution injection of the interspinous ligament in a double-blind study of 100 patients [81]. The treated group improved more rapidly, based upon pain relief and an ability to resume work. Goebert observed 72% good results using the technique, while Winnie et al. suggested that steroid injection was responsible for pain relief and improved work status in 80% of his patients after six months of follow-up study [82,83]. The efficacy of epidural injection is also confirmed by Yates, who presented evidence which showed injection of local anaesthetic and steroids to be more effective than saline or local anaesthetics injected individually [84].

Others have challenged these notions, citing epidural injection to be of short term value at best. For instance, White showed that in 20% of cases reviewed, patients were not cured because of inaccurate needle placement [85]. Of the 84% that did have short term relief, pain reduction fell to just 34% of the group six months after treatment. Green et al. used steroid injection in a sample of 60 back pain patients and found improvement in 30% at a one-year follow-up [86]. A major distinction in pain reduction was seen between acute and chronic patients; those who had suffered back pain for more than three months did much worse than the acute cases.

Klenerman et al. conducted a randomized trial of lumbar epidural injections for the treatment of sciatic pain [87]. The 63 patients were allocated between four injection modalities: 20 ml normal saline solution, 80 mg Depo-medrone in 20 ml normal saline, 20 ml 0.25% bupivacaine solution in saline, and a placebo of needling the interspinous ligament with no injection. All of the participants were suffering from unilateral sciatica of six months or less duration. Overall, 75% of the patients improved or were cured, with no significant differences in rate of recovery among the four treatment groups. Considering the significant number of patients successfully treated by needling of the interspinous ligament, Klenerman asserts that "it seems likely that the epidural injections administered achieved effect partially as a placebo and partially by virtue of the natural history of the acute sciatic syndrome."

This finding correlates closely to the observations of Swerdlow et al., who noted an identical pain reduction rate of 75%. Bupivacaine with methylprednisolone acetate was compared to lidocaine by Mathews, with all patients injected three times at two week intervals [89,90]. The first assessment of epidural injection at one month showed that 67% of the treated and 56% of the controls had improved upon their six-point visual analog pain scales, the difference not reaching statistical significance. By three months, the treated group was only slightly better off than the controls, with almost no statistical differences between groups. Bupivacaine epidural injection was also analyzed by Berman et al. in a study of the effects of local anesthetics and corticosteriod injection in 367 patients with leg pain [91]. The study was a restrospective evaluation with an average follow-up period of 21 months, and therefore lacked a control population for ideal treatment comparison. All patients had undergone a minimum of two weeks of conservative therapy (average of two months), which included bed rest, analgesics, anti-inflammatory drugs and physical therapy. Each patient was given 10 ml of 0.5% bupivacaine, 92% of the patients received 100 mg of methylprednisolone and 8% received 100 mg of hydrocortisone.

The results were graded by four classifications. "Excellent" results reflected complete pain relief, no work restrictions and no need for further treatment. Patients with "good" results had complete or near complete relief or pain and minimal work restrictions, while some additional outpatient conservative treatment was necessary. At the initial three month follow-up, 87% of those patients with subacute pain and no prior surgical history (Group I) had excellent or good results, while 13% of this group had fair or poor results. Patients with chronic pain without surgical history (Group II) demonstrated 76% excellent to good results, 24% achieving fair to poor results. Those patients with chronic pain and a prior history of lumbar surgery (Group III) presented with 50% excellent to good results, and 50% fair to poor results. One year after the initial injection, pain relief was still apparent but had diminished in magnitude. Group I patients had 69% excellent to good results, Group II had 63% and Group III had only 34%. Adverse side effects were seen in 6.3% of the cases, most notably 10 cases of transient hypotension, 5 cases of voiding difficulty, and 4 cases of severe paresthesia. There were no systemic side effects from the steroids. It was concluded that the pivotal determinant influencing the outcome of injection was a history of previous lumbar surgery. Patients with positive myelograms, EMGs or reflex or motor deficits were also likely to benefit from injection.

Chymopapain

Chymopapain is the most common type of chemonucleolytic treatment currently available, and certainly the most controversial. Its origin is traced to 1963, when Dr. Lyman Smith demonstrated that small doses of the extract of papaya latex dissolved nucleus pulposus in rabbits. Larger doses were found to dissolve the annulus fibrosus as well. By 1975, almost 17,000 patients suffering from lumbar disc herniation had been treated with this enzyme [93]. Fisher explains the rationale for chymopapain injection in this way: "An enzyme specific to one or more components of the disk should be capable of dissolving those components in the matrix of the nucleus pulposus, thus relieving the pressure of herniated material on nerve endings and spinal nerve roots and alleviating the symptoms caused by such pressure." [94]

Many attempts have been made to assess the safety and efficacy of chymopapain in the treatment of patients with a herniated lumbar disk who were candidates for laminectomy. Even so, until this decade, there remained no definitive assessment of chymopapain's efficacy in lumbar disk disease based on a carefully conducted, randomized, controlled trial. If a recent survey of neurosurgeons by the American Association of Neurological Surgeons is any barometer of opinion about chemonucleolysis, it appears that chymopapain has been uniformly rejected by neurosurgeons [95]. In this 1984 poll, over half (52%) of the 858 neurosurgeons responding to the questionnaire had discontinued the procedure because it was not efficacious (42%) or the risks were too great (33%). Additionally, 87% of the surgeons believed chymopapain to be less efficacious than surgery, while only 1% believed it to be a more effective treatment.

Recent studies on chymopapain do not reflect such a consensus. Many claim that chymopapaine is no more effective than saline, and considerably more dangerous. Other studies within the last five years report good to excellent treatment of approximately 70 to 80% of those patients consenting to intradiscal injection, documenting a superiority to placebo, discectomy and laminectomy. These authors emphasize the role that chemonucleolysis can play in selective cases of disc herniation, the lower cost, faster recovery, and significantly reduced potential for arachnoidal, intraneural and muscular scarring when compared with surgery. For example, in a double-blind study of 60 patients with unilateral sciatica, Fraser [93] found chymopapain injection to provide complete pain relief in 63% of those treated, versus 27% success with saline-injected patients [93]. Six months later, 80% of chymopapain patients presented satisfactory results, compared with 57% of the control group. The author concluded: "In all of the parameters measured, there was a trend for patients treated with chymopapain to do better than those treated with saline".

A similar success rate is described by Benoist et al, who observed satisfactory relief in 90 of 120 patients [96]. Disc sequestration (free-floating fragments of bone and disc within the spinal canal) and segmental stenosis were the major cause of failure in this study, a probable contraindication to treatment confirmed by several other investigators. Unfortunately, the diagnosis of sequestration can be difficult, even with the most advanced imaging techniques. Regarding spinal stenosis, the disc space shrinkage following chemonucleolysis (seen in 100 of 106 patients) may enhance lateral or foraminal stenosis by the drastic reduction in disc height, creating a bony entrapment.

In another randomized double-blind study Javid et al. documented a 73% success rate in 55 patients, compared with 42% for 53 placebo-treated patients [97]. The authors document the deteriorating effects of the placebo, whereas the chymopapain patients maintained relief from pain over several months. This relief was not without side-effect. Fully 49% of the chymopapain-treated patients experienced back spasm, back ache or other adverse reactions. The authors suggest that treatment should not be judged ineffective even if such reactions linger for two or three weeks, as they did in nearly one-third of all those treated who ultimately attained positive results.

Concern over these hazards has drawn attention to the safety of chemonucleolysis. Fisher gives an account of a study which compares the safety of chymopapain to surgery [94]. Of 13,200 treated patients, 401 instances of chymopapain-induced complications were reported, in addition to a mortality rate of 0.06% and a hypersensitivity reaction estimate of 1% to 1.5%. Surgery was found to have considerably higher risks, with a 6% incidence of complications, a mortality rate of 0.17% and a 6% recurrence rate.

The opponents of chymopapain claim these numbers are misleading and irrelevant. They believe that the higher failure rate, adverse tissue reactions, potentially severe neurologic damage, and a 1% to 2% anaphylaxis rate that are associated with treatment do not justify its role as the last step in conservative therapy. Additionally, severe muscle spasm and back pain, combined with the high incidence of reoperation give the drug no economic advantages [98]. The following studies demonstrate success ratios that are every bit as compelling as the prior findings advocating chemonucleolysis, the fundamental difference being an overwhelming statistical advantage of surgical treatment over injection.

Among the more conclusive reports is one by Norton, which evaluated a population of 105 worker's compensation claimants [99]. Of the 61 cases treated with chymopapain, only 28% of them achieved satisfactory results, versus 59% of those who underwent surgical discectomy. Not only did the surgery group enjoy twice the success rate, but in a calculation of the cost to produce a satisfactory result when failure costs are included, surgery was also shown to be less than half the cost of chymopapain ($49,000 versus $128,000). This result compares favorably with the experience reported by Nachemson [103], and is further validated by Shields [101], who puts the average cost of successful chemonucleolysis at $143,000.

A different experiment by Day et al., attempted to sort the test groups into those units that would yield the most favorable result, selecting out common factors perceived to inhibit recovery (like prior compensation claims) [98]. Of 140 patients analyzed and equally distributed between discectomy and chemonucleolysis, 51% of those treated with chymopapain had an unfavorable result overall, compared with an 80% overall success rate for surgery. When the two groups were restructured to compare the most favorable subgroups, the authors were "unable to isolate any chymopapain subgroup that compared favorably with an open procedure. The best possibilities offered to the chymopapain group did not exceed 70% success, compared to the 95% for surgery". In the opinion of the authors, the ideal candidate for chymopapain has yet to be determined.

Yet there are those who believe otherwise, arguing that injection of the enzyme can be effective in the treatment of select lumbar disc conditions. Bridging the gap between those camps advocating or denouncing the procedure, Postacchini et al. discuss the merits of using the preoperative clinical pattern and size of the herniation to screen patients most suitable for chemonucleolysis[101]. By distinguishing three levels of nerve root compression and herniation size, it was discovered that the results of chymopapain treatment in patients having large herniations were significantly inferior to those of surgery. Satisfactory results were seen in 50% of the injected patients, and 89% of the surgery group. However, the enzyme was much more effective on small herniations with low and medium nerve root compression, having a success rate of 100% and 82%, respectively. The authors conclude: "The current study appears to indicate that the rate of satisfactory outcomes and the rapidity with which they are obtained are inversely proportional to the size of the disc herniation." It is their opinion that chymopapain is the treatment of choice for the small disc herniation.

Physical Therapy

Physical therapy is a conservative approach to back pain that utilizes a variety of techniques. Several modalities within the physical therapy regimen have already been elaborated upon in this chapter, including TENS, acupuncture, traction and bracing. This section will address other modalities, including short wave diathermy, ultrasound, soft tissue massage and muscle strengthening exercises. Each treatment will be discussed in terms of therapy objective and clinical efficacy.

Heat can be administered either superficially to surface tissue or delivered directly to the muscles. Proponents claim both techniques are useful because they reduce pain, raise the pain threshold, and reduce muscle spasm and joint stiffness. Examples of superficial heat include hot packs, hydrocollators, infrared radiation or heating pads. Diathermy and ultrasound are considered deep heating modalities, as they are capable of transmitting heat through the subcutaneous tissue enveloping the muscles. Diathermy has lost considerable popularity among therapists because it has no major advantage over superficial heat in low back treatment. Ultrasound generates heat via a high frequency sound generator which agitates molecules. While the use of ultrasound remains well established in clinical usage, many physicians believe the modality is no more effective than other varieties of deep heat. As far as low back therapy is concerned, Helfet suggests ultrasound is only effective in the treatment of superficial scarring, fibrous tissue, and sprained ligaments and tendons [102]. Jayson recommends this modality for pain relief of trigger points, with treatment usually consisting of 20-minute sessions 2 to 3 times a week for 2 to 3 weeks [103].

Superficial massage is largely without specific benefit to the low back patient other than inducing a pleasant sensation of relaxation. However, vigorous cross-friction administered to defined and palpable structures (e g posterior sacroiliac ligaments) permits the breakdown of minor adhesions, thereby allowing greater local vascularity [102]. Other physicians claim massage (as well as heat) may make the patient feel better temporarily, but does nothing to speed the resolution of the symptoms. Consistent with the perspective of the orthopedic community is the following statement by Macnab [104], a highly distinguished surgeon: "To request massage is no more than using the physical therapy department as a medically approved body rub parlor" [104].

Exercise is perhaps the most valuable component of physical therapy. There are two major schools of exercise therapy for low back pain. Flexion exercises are most widely prescribed, emphasizing the stretching of tight posterior muscles and ligaments and avoidance of lumbar spine extension. This treatment is based upon the assumption that flexion of the posterior longitudinal ligament and posterior annular fibers help push the contents of a bulging disc anteriorly away from compressed nerve and dural structures. Proponents of flexion exercise also believe that facet joint encroachment of the posterior foramina is reversed, reducing nerve root compression. The counterpart to flexion therapy is extension exercise. Advocates of extension exercise claim that when the lumbar spine is extended, the posterior vertebral end-plates are approximated and can act as a wedge to squeeze any posterior bulging nuclear material anteriorly, reducing the posterior aspects of a bulging disc upon adjacent nerve roots.

In either case, flexion and extension exercises attempt to create a "corset of muscle" to redirect weight from the discs, ligaments and other structures responsible for pain [105]. Additionally, such exercise therapy is seen as beneficial to improving the mobility of the spine. Yet Nachemson argues that these traditional exercise programs may do more harm than good: "Many of these exercises increase the load of the lumbar spine to such an extent that it reaches magnitudes as high as those measured in standing and leaning forward with weights in the hands. There is general agreement that such positions should be avoided by back patients!" [106]

Instead, Nachemson recommends isometric exercises for the abdominal and quadriceps muscles, rather than for back muscles. Two different controlled studies by Kendall et al. have demonstrated that such exercises alone or in conjunction with traction gave better clinical results than ordinary flexion and extension programs [107,108]. Rather than conditioning the back muscles, Nachemson argues that increasing intra-abdominal pressure through an isometric abdominal exercise program is more effective in reducing the load of the lumbar spine.

Empirical evidence concerning the efficacy of physical therapy is limited because most research has relegated therapy to control group status, incorporating such treatment to serve only as a backdrop to prove the legitimacy of other conservative modalities. In addition to some of the studies listed in the Low Back School section of Chapter One, a report by Lidstrom et al. is one of the few studies to analyze the effectiveness of physiotherapy in terms of two types of therapy programs [105]. Sixty-two patients with similar symptoms of sciatic pain radiating down one leg for more than one month's duration were randomly allotted to one of three groups. Group I received conventional treatment consisting of hot packs, massage, mobilization and back strengthening exercises. Group II received mostly intermittent pelvic traction, in addition to isometric training of the abdominal and hip extensor muscles. Group III was treated with hot packs and rest. The effectiveness of Group II treatment was significantly greater than the other groups. Of the 30 patients who were receiving analgesics before treatment, 7 in Group I and 4 in Group 4 were still taking them, whereas Group II (traction with isometric exercise) showed a dramatic reduction in the consumption of analgesics after treatment, from nine patients before treatment to none after treatment. This finding tends to support Nachemsons's opinion regarding the efficacy of isometric exercise used alone or in conjunction with intermittent traction.

Surgical Treatment

Introduction

The United States has the highest number of back surgeries in the world, the overwhelming majority related to disc pathology. In 1982, approximately 200,000 discs were excised. Between the period 1975 to 1980, 700 disc procedures per million inhabitants were performed annually in the US, compared to 540 procedures per million in Canada, 260/million in Norway, 180/million in Sweden and 80/million in Great Britain [109]. The literature demonstrates widely varying success rates for back surgery, ranging from 19% to 95%. Many believe that the only group of patients that profit from surgery are those who have herniated discs with definite nerve root involvement [110,111]. As discussed in the preceding chapters, this group is only a minute percentage of the overall back pain population, approximately 1% to 2% of all low back pain cases. At present, surgical treatment is limited to two primary objectives: decompression of neural tissues, and fusion (arthrodesis) of an unstable or arthritic vertebral segment. Lumbar spine surgery is generally directed toward the restoration of nerve root function or the relief of intractable nerve root and mechanical pain.

Since most of the literature implicates poor criteria in patient selection as the most common cause of surgical failure, it is important for the reader to understand the indications for surgical intervention. The following treatment sequence outlines a model of decision-making for surgery, proposed by Rothman as a traditional pre-operative program [112]. Before surgery is initiated, the acute back patient should be treated in a conservative manner, unless there is significant or deteriorating muscle weakness (as in cauda equina syndrome or foot drop). If the patient has not improved with this regimen after four to six weeks, the surgeon must determine whether the predominant symptom is surgically treatable. For instance, the distinction between mechanical and non-mechanical sciatica is tremendously important – the latter condition may respond to epidural steroid injection, while the former may only respond to surgical intervention. Rothman suggest that the spinal surgeon is well-advised to use the following logic: "There should be an anatomic lesion you can remove surgically – a ruptured disc or possibly spinal stenosis. There should be a complaint of pain in the leg of the patient. And there should be an objective test, such as the straight leg raising test, to tie these symptoms together. Alternatively, if it is a disc hernia, instead of a complaint of pain there should be a neurologic finding... When those three groups intersect, you will have excellent results; when they do not, you will have marginal results... If one factor is absent, you are going to drop down to a success rate of about 65%. If two are absent, you are in big trouble."

Sprangfort concluded that the the single most important condition predicting a successful outcome among 2,504 lumbar discectomies was the degree of disc herniation [113]. It was observed that most patients without herniation did not benefit from lumbar disc surgery, although 38% of patients who underwent negative exploration experienced placebo benefit with relief of sciatic symptoms. Implicit in this finding is the belief that the main objective of lumbar disc surgery should be to discover and remove an extruded nucleus pulposus. Jackson [114] has found that while roughly 60% of patients should have an excellent result, 10% will fail to respond or develop worse symptoms after the operation.

Samplings from others revealed a surgical failure rate in excess of 15% in the United States. The most common source of failure in lumbar disc surgery, according to Frymoyer, is poor patient selection, in that the cause of pain was uncertain, the surgery was performed because of a dominant symptom of low back pain instead of sciatica, or the patient had a psychological state associated with poor results [19]. "Patients at particular risk for poor outcomes can be identified on the basis of Waddell's signs (physical findings suggesting a behavioral disturbance), an abnormal pain drawing (that is, the indication by the patient of pain that is not anatomically plausible), pending workman's compensation claims, and psychological tests showing hysteria, hypochondriasis, and somatization."

Beyond the psychological realm, there are several physiologic circumstances that are detrimental to surgical outcome. In some instances, the sciatica or back pain may be due to a disc prolapse at a different level than the one excised, or because of stenosis in the root canal caused by facet impingement. Scar tissue formation has been known to hinder the progress of many post-surgical cases, as it can develop around the root, reproducing the pressure of the prolapsed disc, or even result in arachnoiditis. Finally, disc excision does not rule out the possibility of future disc herniation at the same or another level.

The remainder of the chapter will address the effectiveness of three types of surgical techniques: Discectomy, Percutaneous nuclectomy, and Fusion.

Discectomy

Discectomy is performed exclusively to decompress the nerve root, hence it is most often used in cases of sciatica. A term used to describe a variety of different surgical procedures designed to excise a degenerated or herniated disc, discectomy is a generic "umbrella" that includes laminotomy (partial removal of the lamina), laminectomy, monosegmental interlaminar fenestration, bisegmental fenestration, bilateral interlaminar fenestration, trisegmental disc removal, flavectomy, and hemilaminectomy. Conventional discectomy is usually performed using an intralaminal approach. According to Pheasant et al. there is only one absolute indication for lumbar disc excision: a catastrophic or progressive neurologic problem that may include increasing motor weakness and loss of bowel or bladder function [115]. All other indications for discectomy tend to be somewhat subjective and relative, based upon such factors as the failure of conservative therapy, or confirmed CT or myelographic abnormality with pain. In addition to catastrophic neurologic problems, Spengler lists three other neural pathologies as indications for discectomy: 1. Objective evidence of increasing impairment of root conduction, despite complete bedrest; 2. Severe sciatic pain, associated with root tension, that persists or increases despite four weeks of complete bedrest; and 3. Recurrent incapacitating episodes of sciatic pain with evidence of root tension, or impairment of root conduction, or both [116].

On the basis of several long-term studies, surgeons can point with pride to findings demonstrating surgical treatment to be more effective than conservative treatment for the carefully selected patient, at least in the short run. From the outset, the reader should note that in at least two of the studies listed below, long term analysis allowing ample opportunity for the natural history of back pain to run its course demonstrates no meaningful differences between either treatment modality. For instance, a retrospective study by Hakelius evaluated 583 patients with unilateral L5 or S1 sciatica [117]. Ninety-three percent had received an initial two-month trial of rest and corset brace. Among those patients with myelographically proven herniated discs, more of the surgically treated group reported improvement at two months following initiation of therapy than did the conservatively treated group (97% versus 89%). At a six month follow-up, no significant differences were found. It was also revealed that during the average follow-up period of over 7 years, the conservatively managed group reported more low back pain (71% versus 48%), more residual sciatica (61% versus 44%), more recurrent sciatica (20% versus 10%), and more time lost from work.

A similar pattern was reported by Weber in controlled study which examined whether surgery actually offered advantages over conservative treatment during a decade-long observation period [118]. During a two-week stay in the hospital, 280 patients with sciatica were divided into three groups. Group I consisted of 126 patients presenting with uncertain indications for surgical treatment, later randomly selected for surgical and conservative treatment. It was on this group that Weber conducted the bulk of his analysis. Group II comprised 67 patients presenting definite indications for surgery, while Group

III included 87 patients who continued conservative treatment, based upon moderate symptoms.

A comparison of the two sub-groups of Group I after one year showed that the results were significantly better in the surgically treated group (55/60 having good or fair results after surgery, versus 52/66 for the conservatively treated). The majority of the conservatively treated patients reporting satisfactory results achieved this degree of comfort within six months, suggesting a sufficient period to decide for or against surgery. After four years of observation, no statistically significant differences were noted, although the tendency to a more favorable outcome of surgical treatment was preserved. At the 10-year final examination, no differences in spinal mobility or pain were shown. Recognizing that 25% of the conservatively treated patients were cured and 36% showed fair improvement, Weber emphasizes the fact that "approximately 60% of the operated patients may have been submitted to an unnecessary surgical procedure... Consequently, if the neurologist or another specialist is in doubt regarding further treatment, the patient with low back pain and sciatica should not automatically be referred to the surgeon. The fact that the immediate prognosis after surgery is better does not alter this view."

While Weber's long-term rate of success for surgically treated patients is impressive, even greater success rates were reported in an earlier version of the same prospective controlled trial [119,120]. A number of disc protrusion cases were managed conservatively and surgically (via discectomy), later compared at a four-year follow-up examination. Results indicated that 65% of those operated upon were in good condition, 27% in fair condition, 8% in poor condition, and none in bad condition. After four years, 63% of the surgically treated and 53% of the conservatively treated were completely relieved of back pain. The corresponding figures for radiating pain were 61% and 77%, respectively.

Bouillet's review of 11 separate surgical trials offers additional evidence of the success of discectomy in demonstrating that 6,429 patients had very good or good post-surgical results [121]. In a series of 560 discectomies analyzed between 2 and 11 years post-operatively, Weir found 45% were completely better, 53% partially better, 2.1% unchanged and 0.2% made worse off [122]. Additionally, 80% had returned to their previous activity, while 20% were functioning at a reduced level. Sparup reviewed 14 different operative series (total of 5,175 patients, average follow-up of 4.5 years) and found 51% cured, 82% fit for work, and 8.5% having experienced a recurrence [123].

Nearly all the current literature reports the efficacy of discectomy in the same, favorable light, making a critical comparison difficult. One of the few distinct examples of a study reporting a less-than-glorious success rate is by Frymoyer et al. who followed 64 patients having had discectomies at least ten years previously [124]. Although results showed that 56% had no back pain, 82%

had returned to work, 75% had a normal work status at time of interview, a more probing analysis of the report yielded a disturbingly different picture. The same study indicated that 9% had constant, severe pain upon follow-up, and 34% had intermittent pain. Perhaps more relevant was Frymoyer's categorization of a satisfactory or unsatisfactory end result. An unsatisfactory results was based on any of the following complaints: constant pain, disability from work because of back or leg symptoms, or a need for a second surgical procedure. Of a group of 78 patients, over one-third were classified as having unsatisfactory results (38%). This is in agreement with Spangfort's analysis of 2,504 patients, where 20% to 45% complained of persistent low back pain, and sciatic pain was found in 23% of the patients. Frymoyer emphasizes that the reported statistics are probably optimistic, since 20% of the patients could not be followed.

There are several explanations for discectomy failure. Recurrence of disc herniation (or some type of nerve root irritation) at the same level, or a new level, is one of the most common complications, a consequence of the collapse of disk thickness. Instability is another problem, especially if the joint is susceptible to torsional failure. For example, it has been calculated that removal of the posterior annulus will reduce torque strength by nearly 50%, and by 70% if the disc is already degenerated. Segmental arachnoiditis can result from the varying exposure of the dura to overlying muscle and raw bone. Abnormal stresses in other joints, and persistent symptoms at the same level are also cause for concern. To put this list in perspective, consider a report on the leading causes of failed disc surgery in 268 patients [125]. Recurrent disc herniation at the same level was responsible for 43% of surgical failure, recurrent disc herniation at a new level (22%), segmental instability (18%), and nerve root scarring (12%).

Microsurgical Discectomy

Through the years, the surgical removal of disc and nuclear material has undergone refinement in an on-going effort to reduce blood loss, dissection of muscle and ligament, and tissue scarring. At the same time, maximization in the identification and removal of herniated disc material and fragments has been a primary objective. A technique known as microsurgical discectomy was consequently introduced as a new alternative to standardized discectomy, promising a more effective method of disc excision with the use of small incisions, magnification, and intense illumination of the operative field, a la arthroscopy. The microsurgical approach is accomplished by a small dissection of muscle, adequate resection of bone, maintenance of epidural fat and the nerve sheaths, meticulous bloodless dissection, and gentle manipulation of the nerve root. There are actually several techniques that utilize these methods, designed to address each of the major categories of pathology, including posterolateral disc herniation, lateral disc herniation, superior (or inferior) articular facet hypertrophy, endplate hypertrophy, and subarticular recess stenosis. All techniques emphasize the minimal removal of diseased tissue, with less morbidity to the patient and earlier rehabilitation. Opponents of the procedure cite a higher rate of recurrent symptoms and reoperation due to missed disc fragments.

Most of the post-operative results recorded in the literature document uniformly high success in pain reduction. Williams reported 98% satisfactory results and only 6 reoperations for recurrent scarring among 530 patients [126]. Cooper [127] reported 88% success in a group of 50 patients, and Goald [128] found 97% of 477 patients to have satisfactory results. Wilson et al. obtained good results in 77 of 80 patients treated by microsurgical discectomy [116]. Spengler analyzed 54 consecutive cases (52 with sequestered disc, 2 with protruded lumbar disc herniation) over a minimum 10-month observation period following lumbar discectomy. Follow-up examination showed that 46 had good results, 8 were fair, and none were poor (made worse). Spengler notes that the success rate would be 96% (56/58) if the criterion of finding objective evidence for nerve root compression at the time of surgery was used.

A retrospective review of 485 consecutive patients by Ebeling et al. revealed an excellent outcome in 39%, good in 34%, satisfactory in 19%, and poor in 9% of the patients [130]. A result was considered satisfactory when the post-operative status with regard to pain was better than the preoperative status. The results were based upon operation of patients with unequivocal radicular symptoms with acute paresis or failed conservative treatment. The post-operative observation period ranged from one to three years. Pain relief and capacity to work were judged to be the two most important criteria in the results. Complete or significant pain relief was achieved in 87% to 91% of the patients. While 74% were rehabilitated to a comparable, pre-surgery working capability, 19% of the patients demonstrated reduced working capability, and 7% were incapable of work. Ebeling remarks: "The results obtainable with microsurgery are attained with the standard technique only by a few groups, probably highly experienced surgeons." An identical success rate of 91% is reported by Thomas et al.[131]. Sixty patients with sciatica were followed for a minimum of 2.5 years after microsurgical treatment. Forty patients (66%) reported no sciatic pain at all, while 25% had only minimal symptoms. Only two patients complained of recurring sciatica.

Percutaneous Discectomy (Nuclectomy)

Percutaneous discectomy offers a number of theoretical advantages over laminectomy in the surgical treatment of lumbar disc herniation and associated radicular pain. The procedure utilizes a tube passed through the retroperitoneal soft tissues and psoas muscle to the lateral border of the disc. Once the tube has been positioned with the aid of a fluroscope, specially lengthened rongeurs or motorized shavers are inserted at a 45 degree angle through the tube to remove disc material in piecemeal fashion. Because the surgical path bypasses the spinal canal, dural sac, articular processes, facet joints, and nerve roots, the approach permits disc decompression in much the same way that chymopapain does, without the potential hazard of anaphylaxis. Consequently, chemical discitis does not occur. In this manner, a reduction of disc volume and pressure is achieved, presumably relieving sciatic pain.

As there is no lumbar incision, percutaneous discectomy avoids the muscle stripping, bone removal, and nerve root retraction that characterizes laminectomy. The epidural space is not violated and the nerve root is not directly manipulated. Furthermore, only a small portion of the spinal nerve is subject to insult. The avoidance of epidural bleeding and secondary scarring may reduce the incidence of increased neurological deficit after operation and late failure caused by arachnoiditis. Minimal tissue-scarring also results in decreased hospitalization, increasing the likelihood of rapid return to work. The incidence of future herniation is unlikely, as the excised nucleus pulposus taken from the surgically-punctured annulus prevents the build-up of intradiscal pressure. Should reherniation occur, the fenestrated "portal" will ensure that prolapsed material is directed away from the neural elements.

There are some disadvantages which limit the usefulness of percutaneous discectomy. The procedure is contraindicated in patients with cauda equina syndrome, very large disc herniations, and in cases where the herniation is no longer contained by the annulus. Damage to major vessels (i e aorta, inferior vena cava) or the bowel located in the retroperitoneal surgical path is a remote possibility. Medial disc herniation is more difficult to excise using the procedure than posterolateral disc herniation. Furthermore, the L5-S1 disc may be difficult to approach.

While only short-term results have been published, the literature appears to view the procedure in a favorable light. Kambin et al. operated using a posterolateral approach upon 50 consecutive patients demonstrating intractable sciatic pain, positive root tension signs, neurological impairment and correlative myelography [132]. After an average follow-up period of 27 months (ranging from 12 to 41 months), the patients were evaluated in accordance with a grading system by Macnab: an excellent outcome indicated that the patient was free of pain, had no restriction of mobility, and was able to return to normal work and activities; a good outcome indicated occasional pain and the ability to return to modified work. Significant relief of sciatica was experienced by 84% of the patients within the first 24 hours post operatively. The average hospitalization period lasted 2.3 days. At the end of the follow-up period, 80% of all patients were rated as good or excellent. None of the patients experienced neurologic deficit, wound infection, or disc space infection postoperatively.

Freidman reported a high efficacy rate among nine patients receiving percutaneous discectomy [133]. All seven patients with clear evidence of radicular pain and corroborative radiographic findings claimed excellent relief of symptoms. A much larger study group of 71 patients with disc herniation (most combined with narrow spinal canal and spondylolisthesis) demonstrated a lower rate of success in a report by Suezawa et al.[134]. In rating the clinical success, the following factors were taken into account: pain, mobility, radicular signs, local symptoms, and ability to work. The results were found to be very good in 18 patients, good in 22, satisfactory in 9, and unchanged in 22 patients. While these results are less impressive, the author notes that surgery was undertaken on patients with a variety of back ailments, not just the classic disc herniation case. Approximately 70% of the patients with only a herniation at one level obtained very good or good results, whereas the patients with disc herniation combined with other causes of pain – spondylolisthesis, spondylolysis, or narrowing of the spinal canal achieved very good or good results in only 30% of such cases. Improvements in percutaneous discectomy continue to be developed. Investigations are currently under way in the use of laser probes which vaporize the disc. Newer motorized shavers with guillotine knives and suction are becoming popular. It appears that success rates for the procedure range between 60% to 80%.

Lumbar Fusion (Arthrodesis)

The primary objective of spinal fusion is to reduce and secure the unstable joint producing the symptoms. The historical development of fusion began in 1911 when Hibbs proposed spine fusion for treatment of progressive, deforming spinal disease [135]. Despite three-quarters of a century of lumbar spinal fusion application to low back pain disorders, this therapeutic modality remains a highly emotional and controversial subject in the neurologic and orthopedic community. According to Sypert, such responses are appropriate given the absence of generally accepted operational definitions of mechanical low back/sciatic pain (aka lumbar, segmental instability) [136]. Even so, the annual incidence of lower lumbar and lumbosacral fusion in the United States has risen from 5.2 per 100,000 in 1979 to 9.9 per 100,000 in 1983, according to data from the National Center for Health Statistics [137].

Careful review of the literature fails to elicit scientifically interpretable data that may be used to determine the patient selection criteria which would maximize the success of arthrodesis. Indications vary from surgeon to surgeon. Moreover, there have been no well-designed prospective clinical studies that rigorously document the specific role of spinal fusion in the treatment of low back disorders, unlike the research on lumbar discectomy. Because of the wide varity of possible indications for lower lumbar fusions, multiple studies would be required. As will be indicated in the following pages, the bulk of data is uncontrolled and retrospective, making accurate extrapolation difficult.

Since lumbar fusion (whether posterolateral, posterior interbody, or anterior interbody fusion), carries substantial risks and complications for the patient, most doctors feel the use of lumbar fusion should occur in low back pain disorders with proven intractable and incapacitating vertebral instability. Others assert that fusion is warranted in cases where there have been multiple previous laminectomies, in younger patients, or with evidence of significant facet arthropathy. Because of the low rate of pseudoarthosis and complications, posterolateral (intertransverse) fusion has become the technique of choice for most lumbosacral fusions by the majority of orthopedic surgeons. As an example, Farfan et al. portrays the classical deployment of spinal fusion in this manner: "The ideal fusion would be appropriate for a joint with instability, and limited to the single injured joint. It would restore torque strength to near normal, correct any deformity at this joint, and fix the joint in the position of function, preferably without the aid of internal fixation [138]." Regrettably, there is no fusion that meets all of these conditions. (Figure 4-1)

One technique considered effective in the treatment of spondylolisthesis and disc degeneration is anterior interbody fusion of the lumbar spine. Raugstad et al. performed surgery on 47 patients using this method, evaluating the results two to six years post operatively [139]. Most of the patients had had pain for one year prior to surgery, while many had been out of work for several years. Of 26 patients suffering from spondylolisthesis, 42% were cured and 35% were made better. This compares with 68% cured and 21% made better for those patients treated for disc degeneration. Among the 45 total patients, about half went back to their previous jobs, 50% of which involved heavy manual work. Twenty-five percent of the study group had to change to lighter work. Anterior fusion gave an acceptable result in 37 of 45 patients.

Van Rens et al. achieved even better results using the same anterior interbody fusion in 24 cases of spondylolisthesis [140]. All had clinical symptoms of instability or vertebral slip. Follow-up ranged from 10 to 17 years post operatively. The results criteria included a subjective questionaire dealing with pain severity during work or social activities. One year after surgery, 21 of the 24 patients had no pain complaints. Ten years post operatively, 20 of the patients had maintained a pain-free status. Based upon these results, the authors suggested that a solid structural bony fusion could be achieved within 4 to 6 months postoperatively in 23 of the 24 patients. As for complications, only one case of pseudoarthrosis was observed; no signs of early deterioration of the segments adjacent to the fused area were noted.

An analysis of the long-term consequences of lumbar fusion by Lehmann141 includes the longest post operative follow-up of any retrospective longitudnal study found in the current literature [141]. The main purpose of the follow-up was to determine the long-term prognosis for patients undergoing lumbar fusion. Sixty-two patients were followed for 21 to 52 years (average 33 years).

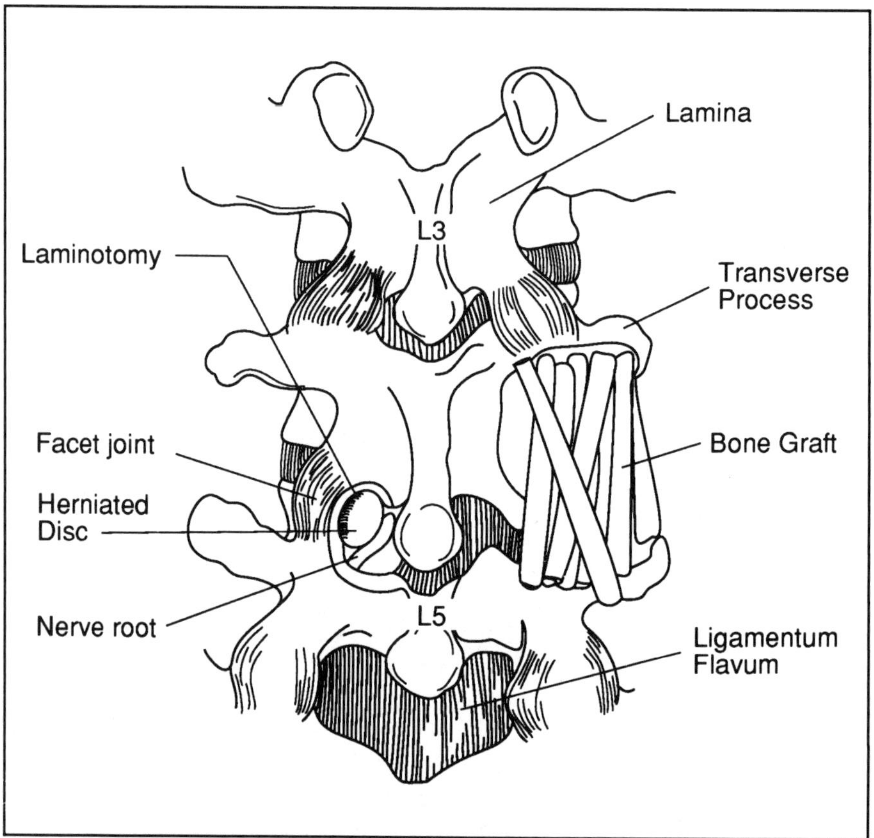

Fig 4-1: This figure illustrates a lumbar transverse process fusion with bone graft strips on the RIGHT side and a laminotomy for disc herniaton on the LEFT side. Normally, the fusion procedure would involve the transverse processes on both sides.

All were operated on before 1964. Although 44% reported that they were currently experiencing back pain, and 57% reported back pain in the last year, 92% indicated that they would have the lumbar fusion again. On a 10-point Visual Analog Scale, the pain index average was 2.33, indicating relatively little pain. Pseudoarthrosis occurred in 30%, and iliac donor-site tenderness was seen in 55%. Nearly half the group (47%) was using some kind of medication (mostly non-narcotic) on a regular basis. Lehmann concludes: "Although patients undergoing lumbar fusion can expect a greater probability of having low-back symptoms in their retirement years than the general population, the evidence reported here suggests that the severity of the symptoms for the majority of patients was not prohibitive."

Sometimes fusion is combined with simple disc excision, the logic being that joint immobilization after a discectomy will drastically reduce pain by preventing intersegmental instability or foramenal stenosis. Yet the literature has been unable to conclusively support this logic. The subject remains a source of constant debate. Frymoyer, for instance, determined that midline spinal fusion offers few benefits in the management of lumbar disc disease, based upon a minimum ten-year retrospective follow-up of 207 patients [142]. A partial laminectomy with simple disc excision was performed on 64 patients, while 143 patients had partial laminectomy, disc excision and posterior midline fusion. There were no differences between the groups with respect to the frequency of back or leg symptoms, or function.

With respect to pain complaints, disability from work, or need for a second surgical procedure, the combined failure rate was 30% for the 166 patients who had an initial fusion. Of the 78 patients who initially did not undergo fusion, 38% were classified as having failed treatment, which is not statistically significant. In patients having fusion, the most common source of failure was pseudoarthrosis of the midline fusion mass, as well as graft donor-site pain. These findings run parallel with the evidence in two other long-term follow-up studies submitted by Barr et al.[143] and Nashold et al.[144], both of which demonstrate a slight but statistically insignificant benefit for combined fusion. Frymoyer writes: "Fusion does not improve long-term results in the treatment of lumbar disc herniation and is rarely indicated."

Tria et al. reached the same conclusion in a retrospective evaluation of two groups of patients surgically treated for herniated nucleus pulposus with a follow-up period from 3.5 to 16 years [145]. The results of each surgery were evaluated on a 100-point system. The average score for 42 laminectomies was 69 points (average score for compensation case = 52), compared with an average score of 70 for the group having laminectomy and fusion. Excellent to good results were demonstrated in 59% of the laminectomies and 64% of the laminectomies with fusion; the difference was judged to be statistically insignificant. However, the reoperation rate of the simple laminectomy group was three times higher than those having laminectomy and fusion.

White et al. reported that when hardware was used to augment the fusion, the results were actually worse than discectomy alone [146]. Sixty-nine patients were divided into two groups, one receiving bilateral lumbar laminectomy and disc excision, the other receiving exactly the same procedure with the addition of an intertransverse fusion with internal fixation. The post operative follow-up average was 4.9 years for the fusion group (38 patients) and 3.7 years for the non-fusion group (31 patients). Significantly, the results of the study can be interpreted with substantially greater confidence than either of the two previous reports. The data is entirely based upon a controlled, prospective study on a matched set of patients, all operated upon by the same surgeon. Both groups had similar age, sex and occupational characteristics.

A successful treatment was expressed in terms of activity level, medication, subjective and objective evaluation. For example, an excellent rating was given to patients who were free of all residual limitations and deficits -- a complete recovery. A good result meant at least a 70% reduction in pain and a return to full activities, sports, and the same job. An excellent or good rating was observed in 71% of patients treated without fusion, and 53% of patients treated with fusion. If fair results are also included, then both groups were 87% successful. The authors respond: "These results would indicate that the fusion with internal fixation does not increase the success (of herniated disc treatment), but in fact diminishes it. Additional time at surgery, blood loss, and potential complications from fusion and internal fixation do not seem warranted." Sypert is even more outspoken in his condemnation of the routine practice of fusion at the time of excision: "There is absolutely no evidence that lumbar fusion improves the results of a well-executed decompressive discectomy in an appropriately selected patient. Given currently available data, the only rational conclusion that can be reached is that the routine addition of lumbar fusion can only add to the morbidity of the treatment" [136].

Summary

The variations in treatment for low back pain may be exceeded only by the number of people who suffer from lumbar disorders. Some would view this plethora of prescriptions as an admission that no single form of therapy is truly effective. Perhaps a more accurate view is that the many causes of low back pain require individualized remedies if the underlying problem is to be cured. Bed rest may be useless for someone with a massive disc extrusion compressing a nerve root. Disc surgery may not work for someone with a muscular back strain. To be most effective, treatment should be carefully correlated with an accurate diagnosis.

For the vast majority of low back problems, conservative measures will not only suffice but will give the most beneficial and least costly result. Rest and time will cure 70% to 80% of back pain problems in just a few days. Overreacting to the very early stages of back pain with too aggressive a treatment program can actually impede the body's healing process.

After the acute phase most patients benefit from exercise and activity in order to regain strength and flexibility. Medication can also be useful. Surgery is reserved for those cases that have failed conservative treatment. But failure to improve is not enough. An intelligently planned approach based on evidence of anatomic pathology should be in place if back surgery is to have a good chance of success. (Figure 4-2)

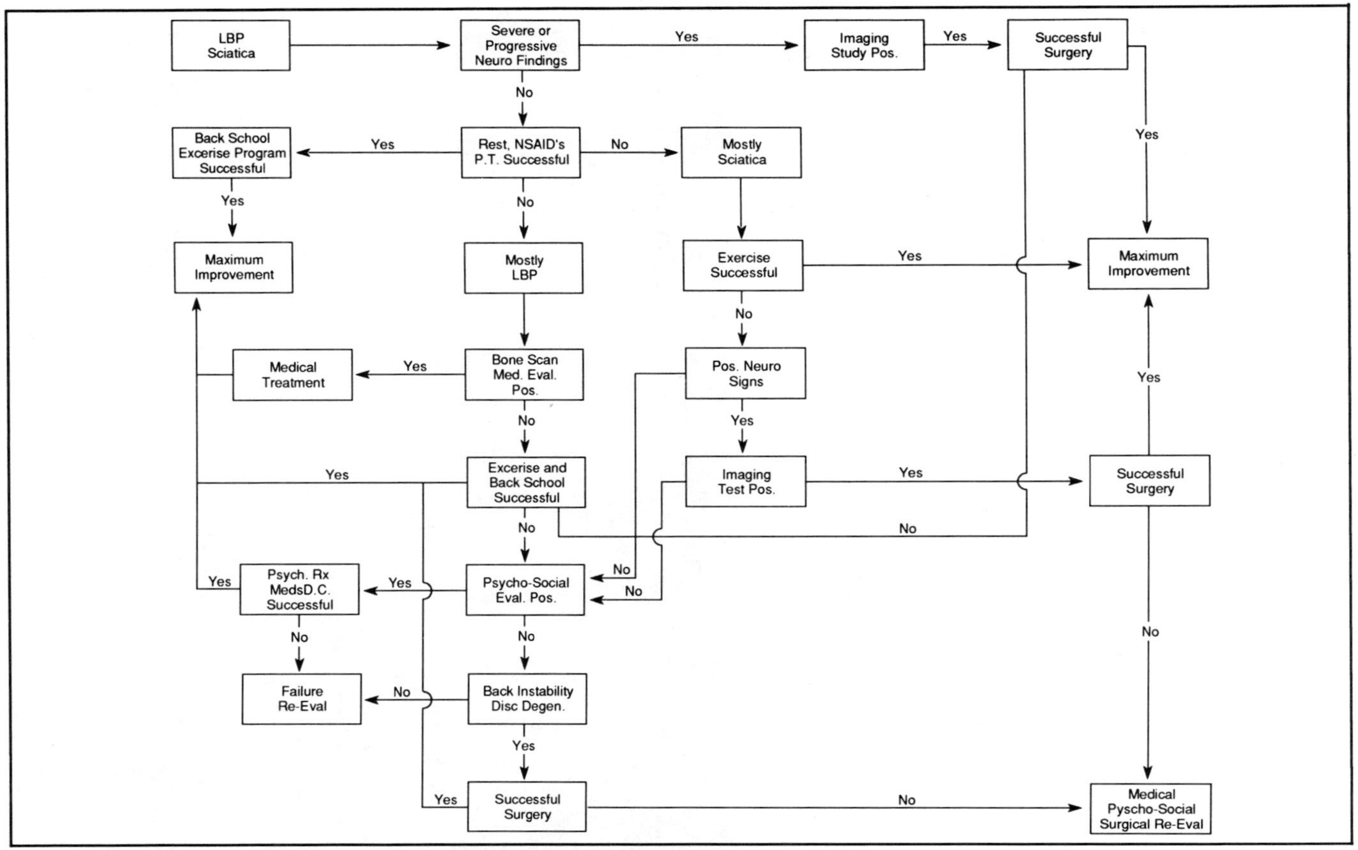

Fig 4-2: A treatment decision tree for low back patients. LBP=low back pain. POS.=positive. NEURO.=neurologic. P.T.=physical therapy. NSAID'S=non-steroidal anti-inflammatory drugs. D.C. MEDS=discontinue medications. PSYCH. Rx=psychiatric treatment. MED. EVAL.=internal medicine evaluation. (modified from Rothman, R.H. and Simeone, F.A.: The Spine, Saunders, 1981.)

References

1. Andersson GJB, Svensson HO, Oden A: The intensity of work recovery in low back pain. Spine 8:880-884, 1983.
2. Editors of Spine Magazine. Chapter 4 – Treatment of activity-related spinal disorders. Spine 12(No. 7 supplement):22-30, 1987.
3. Nachemson A: The load on lumbar discs in different positions of the body. Acta Orthop Scand 36:426, 1965.
4. Rothman R, Simeone FA: The Spine. JB Lipincott, Philadelphia, 1980.
5. Waddell G: A new clinical model for the treatment of low back pain. Spine 12:632-644, 1987.
6. Gilbert JR, Taylor DW, Hildebrand A: Clinical trial of common treatments for low back pain in family practice. Br Med J 291:791-794, 1985.
7. Lindstrom A, Zachrisson M: Physical therapy on low back pain and sciatica -- an attempt at evaluation. Scan J Rehabil Med 2:37-42, 1970.
8. Deyo RA, Diehl AK, Rosenthal M: How many days of bed rest for acute low back pain? A randomized clinical study. N Engl J of Med 315:1064-1070, 1986.
9. Wiesel SW, Rothman RH: Acute low back pain. An objective analysis of conservative therapy. Clin Orthop 143:290, 1979.
10. Nutter P: Aerobic exercise in the treatment and prevention of low back pain. Occup Med: State of the Art Reviews 3(1):137-155, 1988.
11. Bortz WM: The disuse syndrome. West J Med 141:691-694, 1984.
12. Bigos SJ, Battie MC: Acute care to prevent back disability. Clin Orthop 221:121-130, 1987.
13. Heiser T, Jacobs RR, Casey MP: Ambulatory treatment of acute disc herniations with epidural steriod injection. Orthop Trans 8:418, 1984.
14. Fordyce WE, McMahan R, Rainwater G, et al: Pain complaint-exercise perfromance relationship in chronic pain. Pain 10:311-321, 1981.
15. Lewis JW, Cannon JI, Liebeskind JC: Opoid and nonopoid mechanisms of stress analgesia. Science 208:623-625, 1980.
16. Selby DK: Conservative care of the lumbar spine in the elderly. Geriatrics 38(12):42-56, 1983.
17. Nachemson A: Recent advances in the treatment of low back pain. Internat Orthop 9:1-10, 1985.
18. Rothman RH: Decison-making in low back surgery. Bull of the Hosp for Joint Disease Orthop Inst 46(2):93-107, 1986.
19. Frymoyer JW: Back pain and sciatica. New Engl J of Med 318(5):291-300, 1988.
20. Carron H, RE McGlaughlin: Management of Low Back Pain. pp 149-152. PSG, Inc., 1982.
21. Gingras M: A clinical trial of Tofrani in rheumatic pain in general practice. J Int Med Res 4(suppl 2):41-49, 1976.

22. A White: Conservative care. From RG Watkins, JS Collis, Jr. Lumbar Discectomy and Laminectomy - Principles and techniques in spine surgery. Aspen, 1987.
23. Nachemson A, Elfstrom G: Intravital dynamic pressure measurements in lumbar disc. Scand J Rehabil Med (Suppl) 1:5-40, 1970.
24. Finneson B: Low back pain, Lippincott, Philadelphia, PA 1980.
25. Weber H: Traction therapy in sciatica due to disc prolapse. J Oslo City Hosp 23:167-179, 1973.
26. Christie BGB: Discussion on the treatment of backache by traction. Proc R Soc Med 48:811, 1955.
27. Pal B, Mangion P, Hossain MA, Diffey BL: A controlled trial of continuous lumbar traction in the treatment of back pain and sciatica. Br J of Rheumatol 25:181-183, 1986.
28. Mathews JA, Mills SB, Jenkins VM, Grimes SM, Morkel MJ, Mathews W, Scott CM, Sittampalam Y: Back pain and sciatica: Controlled trials of manipulation, traction, sclerosant and epidural injections. Br J of Rheumatol 26:416-423, 1987.
29. Morris JM, Lucas DB, Bresler B: Role of the trunk in stability of the spine. J Bone Joint Surg 43A:327-351, 1961.
30. Million R, Hall W, Nilsen KH, Baker RD, Jayson MIV: Assessment of the progress of the back patient. Spine 7:204-212, 1982.
31. Grew ND, Deane G: Lumbar spinal support orthoses. Oxford Orthopaedic Engineering Centre Annual Report, pp 23-29, 1978.
32. Gregersen GC, Lucas DB: An in vivo study of the axial rotation of the human thoracolumbar spine. J Bone Joint Surg 48A:247-267, 1967.
33. Lumsden RM, Morris RM: An in vivo study of axial rotation and immobilization of the lumbosacral joint. J Bone Joint Surg 50A:1591-1602, 1968.
34. Waters RL, Morris JM: Effects of spinal supports on the electrical activity of muscles of the trunk. J Bone Joint Surg 52A:51-60, 1970.
35. Morris JM, Lucas BD: Physiological considerations in bracing of the spine. Orthop and Prosth Appl, pp 37-44, 1963.
36. Nachemson A, Morris JM: In vivo measurements of intradiscal pressure. J Bone Joint Surg 46A:1077-1092, 1964.
37. Nachemson A, Schultz A, Andersson G: Mechanical effectiveness studies of lumbar spine orthoses. Scand J Rehabil Med 9 (Suppl):139-49, 1983.
38. Schroeder S, Rossler H, Ziehe P, Higuchi F: Bracing and supporting of the lumbar spine. Prosthe and Orthot Inter 6:139-146, 1982.
39. Quinet RJ, Hadler NM: Diagnosis and treatment of backache. Sem Arthr Rheum 8:261-287, 1979.

40. Grew ND, Deane G: The physical effect of lumbar spinal supports. Prosthetics and Orthotics Intl 6:79-87, 1982.
41. Melzack R, Wall PD: Pain mechanisms: A new theory. Science 150:971-979, 1965.
42. Fried T, Johnson R, McCracken W: Transcutaneous electrical nerve stimulation: Its role in the control of chronic pain. Arch Phys Med Rehabil 65:228-231, 1984.
43. Procacci P, Zoppi M, Maresca M: Transutaneous electrical stimulation in low back pain: A critical evaluation. Acupunct & Electro-therapeutics Res Int J 7:1-6, 1982.
44. Indeck W, Printy A: Skin application of electrical impulses for relief of pain. Minn Med 58:305, 1975.
45. Melzack R: Prolonged relief of pain by brief, intense transcutaneous electrical stimulation. Pain 1:357, 1975.
46. Fox EJ, Melzack R: Transcutaneous electrical stimulation and acupuncture: Comparison of treatment for low back pain. Pain 2:141, 1976.
47. Melzack R, Jeans ME, Stratford JG, Monks RC: Ice massage and transcutaneous stimulation: Comparison of treatment for low back pain. Pain 9:207-217, 1980.
48. Thoresteinsson G, Stonnington HH, Stillwell GK, Elveback LR: The placebo effect of transcutaneous electrical stimulation. Pain 5:31-41, 1978.
49. Lehmann TR, Russell DW, Spratt KF, Colby H, Liu YK, Fairchild ML, Christensen S: Efficacy of electroacupuncture and TENS in the rehabilitation of chronic low back pain patients. Pain 26:277-290, 1986.
50. Santeisteban AJ: The role of physical agents in the treatment of spine pain. Clin Orthop, Oct:(179):24-30, 1983.
51. Mendelson G: Acupuncture treatment of chronic back pain. A double-blind placebo-controlled trial. Am J Med 74(1):49-55, 1983.
52. Lee PK, Andersen TW, Modell JH, Saga SA: Treatment of chronic pain with acupuncture. JAMA 232:1133-1135, 1975.
53. Gaw AC, Chang LW, Shaw LC: Efficacy of acupuncture on osteoarthritic pain. New Engl J Med293:375-378, 1975.
54. Moore ME, Berk SN: Acupuncture for chronic shoulder pain. Ann Intern Med 84:381-384, 1976.
55. Edelist G, Gross AE, Langer F: Treatment of low back pain with acupuncture. Can Anaesth Soc J 23:303-306, 1976.
56. Macdonald AJR, Macrae KD, Master BR, Rubin AP: Superficial acupuncture in the relief of chronic low back pain. Annals of the Royal College of Sugeons of England 65:44-46, 1983.
57. Linton SJ, Kamwendo K: Low back schools — a critical review. Phys Ther 67:1375-1383, 1987.

58. Hall H: The Canadian back education units. Physiotherapy 66:115-117, 1980.
59. Kvien TK, Nilsen H, Vik P: Education and self-care of patients with low back pain. Scand J Rheumatol 10:318-320, 1981.
60. Bergquist-Ullman M, Larsson U: Acute low back pain in industry. Acta Orhop Scand (Suppl) 170:1-117, 1977.
61. Dehlin O, Berg S, Andersson GBJ, et al: Effect of physical training and ergonomic counseling on the psychological perception of work and on the subjective assessment of low-back insufficiency. Scand J Rehabil Med 13:1-9, 1981.
62. Lindequist S, Lundberg B, Wikmark R, et al: Information and regime at low back pain. Scand J Rehabil Med 16:113-116, 1984.
63. Gilbert JR, Taylor DW, Hildebrand A, et al: Clinical trial of common treatments for low back pain in family practice. Br Med J (Prac Obs) 291:791-794, 1985.
64. Ljunberg P, Sanne H: Ryggbesvar. Goteborg, Sweden Statshalsan, 1986.
65. Aberg J: Evaluation of an advanced back pain rehabilitation program. Spine 9:317-318, 1984.
66. Lankhorst GJ, van der Stadt RJ, Vogelaar TW, et al: The effect of the Swedish back school in chronic idiopathic low back pain. Scan J Rehabil Med 15:141-145, 1983.
67. Moffett JAK, Chase SM, Portek I, et al: A controlled, prospective study to evaluate the effectiveness of a back school in the relief of chronic low back pain. Spine 11:120-122, 1986
68. Mayer TG, Gatchel RJ, Mayer H, Kishino ND, Keeley J, Mooney V: A prospective two-year study of functional restoration in industrial low back injury. An objective assessment procedure. JAMA 258:1763-1767, 1987.
69. Haldeman S: Spinal manipulative therapy. A status report. Clin Orthop 179:62-70, 1983.
70. Brunarski DJ: Clinical trials of spinal manipulation: a critical appraisal and review of the literature. J Manip Physiol Ther 7:243-249, 1984.
71. Glover JR, Morris JG, Khosla T: Back pain: A randomized clinical trial of rotational manipulation of the trunk. Br J Ind Med 31:59, 1974.
72. Godfrey CM, Morgan PP, Schatzker J: A randomized trial of manipulation for low back pain in a medical setting. Spine 9:301-304, 1984.
73. Tobis JS, Hoehler F: Musculoskeletal manipulation in the treatment of low back pain. Bull NY Acad Med 59:660-668, 1983.
74. Nwuga VCB: Relative therapeutic efficacy of vertebral manipulation and conventional treatment in back pain management. Am J Phys Med 61:273-278, 1982.
75. Doran DML, Newell DJ: Manipulation in treatment of low back pain. A multicentre study. Br Med J 2:161-165, 1975.

76. Sim-Williams H, Jayson MV, Young SMS, Baddeley H, Collins E: Controlled trial of mobilization and manipulation for patients with low back pain in general practice. Br Med J 2:1338, 1978.
77. Hoehler FK, Tobis JS, Buerger AA: Spinal manipulation for low back pain. JAMA 245:1835, 1981
78. Farrell JP, Twomey LT: Acute low back pain: Comparison of two conservative treatment approaches. Med J Aust 1:160-164, 1982.
79. Cappio M: Il trattamento indrocortisonico per via epurale sacrale delle lombosciatalgie. Reumatismo 9:60, 1957.
80. Coomes EN: A comparison between epidural anaesthesia and bed rest in sciatica. Br Med J 1:20-24, 1961.
81. Dilke TFW, Burry HC, Grahame R: Extradural corticosteriod injection in management of lumbar nerve root compression. Br Med J 2:635-637, 1973
82. Goebert HW Jr., Jallo SJ, Gardner WJ, Wasmuth CE: Painful radiculpathy treated with epidural injections of procaine and hydrocortisone acetate. Anesth Analg 40:130, 1961.
83. Winnie AP, Hartman JT, Meyers HI Jr., Ramamurthy S, Barangan V: Pain clinic II: Intradural and extradural corticosteroids for sciatica. Anesth Analg 51:990, 1972.
84. Yates DW: A comparison of the types of epidural injection commonly used in the treatment of low back pain and sciatica. Rheumatol Rehabil 17:181, 1976.
85. White AH, Derby R, Wynne G: Epidural injections for the diagnosis and treatment of low back pain. Spine 5(11)76-86, 1980.
86. Green PW, Burke AJ, Weiss CA, Langan P: The role of epidural cortisone injection in the treatment of discogenic low back prompted for inactivity. Clin Orthop 153:121-125, 1980.
87. Klenerman L, Greenwood R, Davenport HT, White DC, Peskett S: Lumbar epidural injections in the treatment of sciatica. Br J of Rheum 23:35-38, 1984.
88. Swerdlow M, Sayle-Creer W: A study of extradural medication in the relief of the lumbo-sciatic syndrome. Anaesthesia 25:341-345, 1970.
89. Brena SF, Wolf SL, Chapman SL, Hammonds WD: Chronic back pain: electromyographic, motion, and behavioral assessments following sympathetic nerve blocks and placebos. Pain 8:1-10, 1980.
90. Mathews JA, Mills SB, Jenkins VM, Grimes SM, Morkel, et al: Back pain and sciatica: Controlled trials of manipulation, traction, sclerosant and epidural injections. Br J of Rheum 26:416-423, 1987.
91. Berman AT, Garbarino JL, Fisher SM, Bosacco SJ: The effects of epidural injection of local anesthetics and corticosteroids on patients with lumbosciatic pain. Clin Orthop 18:144-151, 1984.

92. Fraser RD: Chymopapain for the treatment of intervertebral disc herniation. A preliminary report of a double-blind study. Spine 7:608-612, 1982.
93. R Fisher: Injection therapy for herniated discs - background and usefulness. Postgrad Med - June, 1984.
94. Watts, C: Chymopapain: is it safe and effective? Results of a 1985 AANS/CNS survey. AANS Newslett 10:1-2, 1985.
95. Benoist M, Deburge A, Heripret G, Busson J, Rigot J, Cauchox J: Treatment of lumbar disc herniation by chymopapain chemonucleolysis. A report on 120 patients. Spine 7(6):613-617, 1982.
96. Javid MJ, Nordby EJ, Ford LT, Hejna WJ, Whisler WW, Burton C, Millett DK, Wilste LL, Widell EH, et al: Safety and efficacy of chymopapain (chymodiactin) in herniated nucleus pulposus with sciatica. JAMA 249:2489-94, 1983.
97. Day AL, Savage DF, Friedman WA, Sypert GW: Chemonucleolysis versus open discectomy: The case against chymopapain. Clin Neurosurg 33:385-396, 1986.
98. Norton WL: Chemonucleolysis versus surgical discectomy. Comparison of costs and results in workers' compensation claims. Spine 11(5):440-443, 1986.
99. Nachemson A, Mooney V, Brown M, et al: Symposium: Chemonucleolysis in the management of herniated lumbar disc. Contemp Orthop 9:97-122, 1984.
100. Shields CB: In defense of chemonucleolysis. Clin Neurosurg 33:397-405, 1986.
101. Postacchini F, Lami R, Massobrio M: Chemonucleolysis versus surgery in lumbar disc herniations: Correlation of the results to preoperative clinical pattern and size of the herniation. Spine 12(2):88-96, 1987.
102. Helfert AJ, Gruebel Lee DM (Eds.): Disorders of the Lumbar Spine. JB Limincott Co. 1978. (Text is misspelled - substitute Helfet for Helpert).
103. Jayson MIV (Ed.): The Lumbar Spine and Back Pain. Churchill Livingston, NY, 1987.
104. Macnab I: Backache. Williams and Wilkins, Baltimore, 1977.
105. Lindstrom A, Zachrisson M: Physical therapy on low back pain and sciatica. Scand J Rehab Med 2:37-42, 1970.
106. Nachemson A: Physiotherapy for low back pain patients - a critical look. Scand J Rehab Med 1:85-89, 1969.
107. Kendall PH, Jenkins JM: Lumbar isometric flexion exercises. Physiotherapy 54:158-163, 1968.
108. Kendall PH, Jenkins JM: Exercises for backache: A double-blind controlled trial. Physiotherapy 54:154-157, 1968.

109. Nachemson A, Bigos SJ: The low back. In: Cruess RL, Rennie WRJ (eds) Adult Orthopaedics, Vol. 2. Churchill Livingstone, New York, p 888.
110. Hoehler FK, Tobis JS: Low back pain and its treatment by spinal manipulation: measures of flexibility and asymmetry, Rheumatol Rehab 21:21-26, 1982.
111. Soderberg L: Prognosis in conservatively treated sciatica. Acta Orthop Scand 25 (Suppl):1-127, 1956.
112. Rothman RH: Decision-making in low back surgery. Bulletin of the Hospital for Joint Diseases Orthopedic Institute 46:93-107, 1986.
113. Sprangfort EV: The lumbar disc herniation: A computer-aided analysis of 2,504 operations. Acta Orthop Scand (Suppl 142):1, 1972.
114. Jackson RK: The long-term effects of wide laminectomy for lumbar disc excision. J Bone Joint Surg 53:609, 1971.
115. Pheasant HC, Dyck P: Failed lumbar disc surgery: Cause, assessment, treatment. Clin Orthop, 164(Apr):93-109, 1982.
116. Spengler DM: Lumbar discectomy: results with limited disc excision and selective foraminotomy. Spine 7(6):604-607, 1982.
117. Hakelius A: Prognosis in sciatica. A clinical followup of surgical and non-surgical treatment. Acta Orthop Scand (Suppl) 129:1-76, 1970.
118. Weber H: Lumbar disc herniation. A controlled, prospective study with ten years of observation. Spine 8(2):131-140, 1983.
119. Weber H: Lumbar disc herniation. A prospective study of prognostic factors including a controled trial, Part I. J Oslo City Hosp 28:33, 1978.
120. Weber H: Lumbar disc herniation. A prospective study of prognostic factors including a controled trial, Part II. J Oslo City Hosp 28:89, 1978.
121. Bouillet R: Traitement des lombociatiques par injection intradiscaled de chymopapaine: Analyse comparative des resultats de la discectomie et de la chemonucleolyse. Acta Orthop Belg 42:101, 1976.
122. Weir B: Reoperation rate follwing lumbar discectomy: An analysis of 662 lumbar discectomies. Spine 5:366, 1980.
123. Sparup KH: Late prognosis in lumbar disc herniation. Acta Rheum Scand (Suppl)3:1, 1960.
124. Frymoyer JW, Hanley E, Howe J, et al: Disc excision and spine fusion in the management of lumbar disc disease: A minimum ten-year follow-up. Spine 3:1, 1978.
125. Frymoyer JW: The role of spine fusion - Question 3. Spine 6(3):284-289, 1981.
126. Williams RW: Microlumbar discectomy. A conservative surgical approach to the virgin herniated lumbar disc. Spine 3(2):175-182, 1978.
127. Cooper DF, Feuer H: Lumbar microdiscectomy. J Indiana State Med Assoc 74(10):674-675, 1982.

128. Goald HJ: Microlumbar discectomy. Follow-up of 147 patients. Spine 3(2):183-185, 1978.
129. Wilson DH, Kenning J: Microsurgical lumbar discectomy: preliminary report of 83 consecutive cases. Neurosurgery 4(2):137-140, 1979.
130. Ebeling U, Reinchenberg W, Reuden HJ: Results of microsurgical lumbar discectomy. Acta Neurochir 81:45-52, 1986.
131. Thomas AMC, Afshar F: The microsurgical treatment of lumbar disc protrusion. Follow-up of 60 cases. J of Bone Joint Surg 69b:696-698, 1987.
132. Kambin P, Brager MD: Percutaneous posterolateral discectomy. Anatomy and mechanism. Clin Orthop 223:145-154, 1987.
133. Friedman WA: Percutaneous discectomy: An alternative to chemonucleolysis? Neurosurgery 13(5):542-547, 1983.
134. Suezawa Y, Jacob HAC, Schreiber A: Percutaneous nucleotomy. An alternative to spinal surgery for lumbar disc herniation. Acta Othop Belg 53:293-299, 1987.
135. Hibbs RA: An operation for progressive spinal deformities. NY Med J 93:1013-1016, 1911.
136. Sypert GW: Low back pain disorders: Lumbar fusion? Clin Neurosurg 33:457-483, 1986.
137. Volinn E: Personal communication to Lehmann TR, Spratt KF, Tozzi JE, Weinstein JN, Reinarz SJ, El-Khoury GY, Colby H: Long-term follow-up of lower lumbar fusion patients. Spine 12(6):99-103, 1987.
138. Farfan HF, Kirkaldy-Willis WH: The present status of spinal fusion in the treatment of lumbar intervertebral joint disorders. Clin Orthop 158:198-214, 1981.
139. Raugstad TS, Harbo K, Hogberg A, Skeie S: Anterior interbody fusion of the lumbar spine. Acta Othop Scand 53:561-565, 1982.
140. Van Rens TJ, van Horn JR: Long-term results in lumbosacral interbody fusion for spondylolisthesis. Acta Othop Scand 53:383-392, 1982.
141. Lehmann TR, Spratt KF, Tozzi JE, Weinstein JN, Reinarz SJ, El-Khoury GY, Colby H: Long-term follow-up of lower lumbar fusion patients. Spine 12(6):99-103, 1987.
142. Frymoyer JW, Hanley EN, Howe J, Kulmann D, Matteri RE: Disc excision and spine fusion in the management of lumbar disc disease. A minimum ten-year followup. Spine 3(1):1-6, 1978.
143. Barr JS, Kubik GS, Molloy MK, et al: Evaluation of end results in treatment of ruptured lumbar intervertebral discs with protrusion of nucleus pulposus. Surg Gynecol Obstet 125:250-256, 1967.
144. Nashold BS, Laine S, Hrubec Z: Lumbar disc disease: A twenty year clinical follow–up study. St. Louis, CV Mosby, 1971.

145. Tria AJ, Williams JM, Harwood D, Zawadsky JP: Laminectomy with and without spinal fusion. Clin Orthop 224:134-137, 1987.
146. White AH, von Rogov P, Zucherman J, Heiden D: Lumbar laminectomy for herniated disc: A prospective controlled comparison with internal fixation fusion. Spine 12(3):305-307, 1987.

CHAPTER 5

Prevention

Introduction

While most facets of low back pain give rise to considerable debate, there is no dispute within the medical community that reduction of low back injury industry must be a major goal. The literature is uniform in a consensus that preventive programs must be aggressively introduced and practiced by both the employee and employer. With backache responsible for over 90 million days of lost work and as much as $40 billion in lost productivity, disability payments, treatment costs, law suits and worker retraining, it is certainly in the interest of both management and the national work force to reduce the epidemic incidence of low back pain. Experts have also placed renewed emphasis on prevention of chronic back problems, where 10% of back patients absorb 80% of the money spent for low back care [1,2].

Prevention is essentially accomplished through the avoidance of acute episodes of trauma (i e heavy lifting or sudden twisting) or chronic repeated episodes of excessive stress (such as vibration). It is generally recognized that a prevention program can be categorized into three basic approaches, as proposed by Dwyer and others[3]. Primary prevention attempts to prevent a disorder before it occurs by instruction in lifting or postural techniques, or ergonomic job design. Secondary prevention attempts to limit the disability caused by a disorder before it becomes symptomatic. Tertiary prevention concedes a back problem as inevitable; therefore it attempts to limit the complications of an established symptomatic disorder and reduce the chance of recurrence. Examples of secondary and tertiary prevention include all of the treatment modalities discussed in the previous chapter. Of the three, primary prevention would appear to be the most direct approach to prevention. It is the first line of defense resisting the onset of back pain.

Unfortunately, the identification of symptomatic and asymptomatic individuals most vulnerable to back pain is difficult. Compounding the difficulty is the extent to which corporations and individuals place greater emphasis on treatment and cure (secondary and tertiary prevention) than on primary prevention. Considering that nearly all back problems will resolve within a few months no matter which treatment is utilized, both parties are mostly interested in the "quick fix" that relieves pain and returns the individual to the work place as soon as possible. In many cases, the end result is that neither the employer nor the employee pays attention to the condition until it recurs as a problem.

Despite these impediments to the design, acceptance and adoption of preventive methods, the emphasis on secondary and tertiary forms of preventive treatment is gradually changing to primary prevention. Corporate America has recognized that it is cheaper to keep employees healthy and on the job than to pay for the cost of back disability, rehabilitation and replacement. One example of this trend is seen in a recent survey of the nation's largest 308 employers, which found that worksite back care programs offered by these companies had increased from 6% in 1979 to 12% in 1983 [4]. Many companies have implemented programs that have successfully reduced worker disability attributed to back pain. This chapter will focus on the three most common methods of primary prevention -- worker selection techniques (pre-employment/placement health screening using x-ray analysis and strength testing), ergonomics (job design), and education/training.

Worker Selection Techniques

Health screening is considered a tool for protecting susceptible workers and preventing the economic consequences of job related injuries and illnesses. Medical criteria are used to select and maintain the workforce. More importantly, screening aids the company in the prediction of which workers are most likely to experience disabling low back injuries. Anatomical and physiological criteria are used to determine if a prospective employee is capable of sustaining varying intensities of physical stress over the duration of a projected time period. If the risk of lumbar injury is judged to to be too high, companies will either reject the applicant for employment or assign him to lighter work. Since back pain is responsible for a great deal of worker absenteeism, particular attention is payed to the condition of the lumbar spine. Back screening programs may combine several criteria, including medical history, clinical examination, radiographic evaluation, strength testing, psychosocial tests, and job rating programs. Each will be discussed in terms of safety in administering the test, reliability in predicting the risk of future low back problems, practicality, and the ethical and legal considerations arising from testing.

Medical Examination

In 1956, the American Medical Association's Council on Occupational Health wrote that preplacement examinations "are made for the express purpose of determining and recording the physical condition of the prospective worker and assignment to a suitable job in which his disabilities, if any, will not affect his personal efficiency, safety, and health, nor the safety of others" [5]. The examination is generally divided into two parts – a physical exam, and a medical history. The physical is designed to identify clinical signs of spinal dysfunction which may indicate future risk, evaluating such things as range of motion and posture. Often times, the examiner is unable to assess the risk of future back pain. Yet the physical can still be valuable under such circumstances because it provides an opportunity to screen for surgical scars and artifacts of invasive procedures as well as providing a base line from which to gauge any future changes in back function.

Many authorities feel that the medical history is the most significant part of the medical examination. An accurate and thorough medical history can be instrumental in predicting future back incidence. The more risk factors that a patient has, the greater the chance for injury or recurrence. For example, Lloyd et al. found that a history of residual leg pain, an injury associated with a fall, lost time in excess of five weeks, and a two or more prior back pain episodes in the injured worker increased the probability of recurrence as the number of such factors increased [6]. In fact, Dillane et al. reported that episodes of future back pain are four times more likely after the initial episode [7]. Of course, the real problem with this method is obtaining an accurate history from the prospective employee. Understandably, the worker is sometimes reluctant to reveal information concerning previous low back pain during examination.

Even with a careful history, the prediction of future back pain is very difficult. Rowe estimated that a thorough history might identify roughly 7% to 8% of young individuals prone to future back problems, based upon an evaluation of 1500 cases of back pain monitored over 20 years [8]. Although the identification rate would have been substantially higher among applicants in older age groups (signs of disease being more frequent and obvious) a hit rate of 8% is not an impressive batting average for the industrial practitioner. Moreover, neither Chaffin [9] or Snook [10] were able to validate the effectiveness of preplacement medical examinations (physical or history) in the identification of workers vulnerable to back pain. What these findings indicate most clearly is that a pre-placement or pre-employment screening process must not rely exclusively on the results of a medical examination, but should be supplemented with a number of screening procedures listed below to obtain a more complete picture of the worker's health – past, present, or future.

Pre-employment x-rays

For most of this century, low back x-rays were one of the most prevalent pre-employment test used to evaluate the risk of back injury. While the heyday of x-ray analysis was in the 1950s and 1960s, it is speculated that one million pre-employment back x-rays are currently administered each year at costs ranging from $7.5 to $60 million. The fundamental assumption of radiography is that back x-ray examination will disclose findings which have prognostic significance and can therefore identify the individual who is likely to develop lumbar disability. More specifically, the proponents of radiologic testing believe that strain or trauma to a radiologically-discovered "vulnerable" back structure could be expected to lead to injury and require a longer recovery time than would the same strain or trauma to a "normal" back. However, the observant reader will recognize this as flawed logic, recalling the various reports in the Etiology chapter that have been unable to confirm any differences in reported back pain among groups of symptomatic and asymptomatic individuals with regard to several structural disorders including spondylolysis, spondylolisthesis, spinal stenosis, transitional vertebrae and spina bifida. Additionally, it was also noted in the Diagnosis chapter that radiography is characterized by high rates of false positive and negative evidence, with limited sensitivity and specificity. The "accuracy" of x-ray interpretation, except in cases of developmental defects, fractures or overt disease, is not consistent among different medical observers. There is considerable variability between and among radiologists, orthopedic surgeons, and neurosurgeons in the interpretation of findings.

For example, studies by Rowe have shown that only 10% of 1500 subjects subsequently developing back pain over a 20 year period could have been identified using x-ray analysis as an adjunct to a careful history and physical examination [11,12]. Nachemson [13] found that only one lumbar x-ray in 2500 revealed an unexpected abnormality, while Scavone [14] observed that only one x-ray in eight provided information not revealed in the history or physical exam. Friedman [15] reported that only 20% of 100 healthy soldiers had normal radiographs of the lumbar spine, while Ford [16] found only 7.3% of 1600 x-rays could be interpreted as perfectly normal! Separate studies by Splithoff [17] and Fullenlove [18] demonstrated that congenital defects among symptomatic and asymptomatic groups were equal.

As the history of radiographic screening indicates, it took many years to dispel the widely accepted notion of a correlation between structural deviation and present or future lumbar back pain. Beginning in the early 1920s, reports began appearing about congenital abnormalities such as spondylolisthesis and the increased probability of injury and prolonged recovery. Many asserted the linkage between various bony anomalies and symptomatic conditions, triggering the utilization of radiographs in industry to screen out job applicants with defects. By the end of World War II, many in industry became convinced that radiographic screening could be effectively deployed in an effort to trim disability expenditures. In 1947, Stewart reported that the use of x-rays in screening stevedores had reduced back related disability by 82% [19]. In 1952, Marsh [20] reported a marked decrease in the number of back injuries after instituting a program of pre-employment back radiography, while McGill [21] reported in 1968 a reduction in industrial back claims from $66,000 to $4,400 over a two-year period after the introduction of a pre-employment back program.

Unfortunately, all studies of the predictive ability of preplacement spine films suffer methodological problems as a result of their retrospective nature. Indeed, the ultimate experiment to test the efficacy of this procedure – a randomized controlled trial – has not yet been done. Most of the research that has demonstrated a positive association between structural anomaly and disability has at most indicated that those with defects may have an increased severity, but not an increased incidence of back pain. Runge, for example, found that defects could not predict the incidence of back injuries in a male factory population followed from 1951 to 1956 [22]. However, he did find that three defects increased the duration of work loss. Disc space "abnormality" resulted in 1.43 times longer work loss than observed in "normals". Spondylolisthesis was associated with 1.65 times longer work loss, and previous surgical intervention lengthened work loss by a factor of 5.8. Kosiak reported a major reduction in both the frequency and severity of back injury among 296 plant employees after a pre-employment x-ray screening procedure was adopted; back related absenteeism was reduced from 1500 days in 1960 to only 79 days in 1966, while the workforce increased by 30% and manhours by 60% over the same period [23]. It was concluded that abnormal x-rays would not have predicted the incidence of back pain but might have predicted severity. Even more persuasive results were observed by Connell in an assessment of uranium miners with confirmed x-ray defects [24], compared to miners with no defects. The 343 patients with alleged back disorders lost an average of 34 days of work per patient, while the 687 "healthy" miners missed 18 days. Likewise, the duration of treatment for miners with anomalies was 61 days, compared with 39.5 for those without structural disorder.

A more recent study by Leggo et al. supporting the legitimacy of pre-employment back x-rays evaluated the effectiveness of a back x-ray program for the state traffic officers of the California Highway Patrol [25]. Back injuries in the last two groups of officers appointed before pre-employment lumbar x-rays were adopted were compared to the first two groups which passed the radiographic criteria. As a result of the new medical criteria, the number of back injuries was reduced 12.1%, as well as a decrease of 80.6% in the time lost due to injury. Injuries dropped from 19 per million to 17 per million manhours worked, but the time lost dropped from 299 to 58 days per million manhours. Leggo calculated lost time savings as $141,080 per million manhours worked. The author does note that other factors besides the x-ray program may have favorably influenced the back injury rate.

What is one to make of this bewildering array of documented evidence? On the one hand is the apparent lack of association between structural disorder and symptomatic back pain, while on the other hand excellent results have been documented by companies utilizing that same relationship as criteria for employment. How can such radical differences be reconciled? One explanation is proposed by Montgomery, who asserts that the concept of pre-employment back x-rays occurred during a period when safety programs were receiving extraordinary attention [26]. During the period 1926 to 1961, a four-to-five-fold drop in the frequency and severity of accidents is documented by National Safety Council data [27]. Hence, the extent to which back x-rays reduced disability is confounded by the effects of other safety measures designed to reduce accidents. Only one study attempted to correct for the potential inherent biases of other interventions. That paper showed no improvement in back pain incidence or back-related work loss time resulting from the use of preplacement x-rays [28].

By the late 1960s and 1970s, a number of articles in the literature on pre-employment radiography could no longer substantiate the claims made over the previous fifty years regarding structural disorder, back pain, or disability reduction in industry. For instance, a four-year evaluation by Redfield compared the injury rates of workers assigned to job tasks of varying physical intensity based upon lumbar x-ray defects [28]. Those employees who demonstrated the most structural stability were assigned to a group of "high risk" moderate and heavy physical labor, whereas structurally weaker employees were selected for "low risk" clerical or administrative work. Results indicated that the 209 "high risk" employees had an injury rate only half that of the 1,992 "low risk" workers! The injury rates of the high and low risk groups were 32.5 and 62.3 per thousand, respectively. However, the short follow-up period (average of 24 months) and high drop-out rate precludes any definite conclusions.

In a considerably longer-term analysis, Gibson et al. compared the incidence of low back pain among two groups of steelworkers hired before (634 employees) and after (534 employees) the introduction of back x-rays into an otherwise identical pre-placement medical examination [29]. Each group was followed for twelve years. There was no statistically significant difference between the two groups relative to individuals requiring modified work or lost time. In the prescreen group, 24 individuals lost an average of 52.4 days, while in the post-screen group 20 individuals lost an average of 100.3 days. Furthermore, an evaluation of the drop-outs of the study showed no significant difference between the groups with respect to incidents, or individuals requiring modified work or lost time. Significantly, the negative effects of screening are distorted by the fact that two employees accounted for 49% of the total lost time, indicating the dangers of disproportionate "averaging."

The rejection of qualified applicants based upon radiographic criteria is cause for concern. Rates of disqualification range from 7% to 40% of all prospective employees, many eliminated needlessly who would never have lost time to back disability. For some, future employment and even insurability could be jeopardized by radiographic screening. There may be a significant risk of adverse effects from "labelling," where refusal for employment at one plant may influence hiring decisions another plant. To put this in perspective, consider the experience of the Missouri Pacific Railroad. The company screened 20,000 applicants and rejected about 8,000 (40%) of them based upon x-ray results. According to the calculations of Rockey et al30, 60% of those rejected applicants would never have lost work time to back injury, while 23% of those presenting "normal" spine film would have lost-time injuries [30]. Thus, of the 8,000 disqualified by the railroad, 4,800 of these able-bodied applicants could have sustained employment without significant back pain. Whether or not such a selection process constitutes discrimination or breaches ethics codes is still being disputed in the courts. Indeed, hiring decisions based solely on spinal x-rays do not meet the requirements of the Equal Employment Opportunity Commission, which has ruled that screening must meet the standard of "job relatedness" and not discriminate against those with "perceived handicaps."

What is not contested is the safety implications of routine radiographic screening. Morris writes: "Low back x-rays are the largest single contributor to gonadal irradiation in the United States, which could increase the risk of irradiation-caused diseases by up to 25% (based upon data from the US National Research Council, 1973)." The risk of exposing a woman with an unsuspected pregnancy to unnecessary x-rays can increase the fetal risk of childhood leukemia between two-and ten-fold. The conclusion is that "low back x-rays should always be considered a potential health risk, and any unnecessary use should be discouraged." The remark is echoed by the American Occupational Medical Association, who recommend that low back x-rays "should never be performed in a routine manner and should always be preceded by a careful history and physical examination with special attention to the back. The principal justification for preemployment lumbar spine x-rays is the evaluation of existing disease" [31]. Similar sentiments are expressed by the editor of the Journal of the Canadian Association of Radiologist: "As radiologists we must individually and collectively do all we can to stop the ill-advised practice of routine pre-employment lumbosacral radiographs. It is a practice to be condemned" [32].

Ultrasound

A few researchers have proposed an alternative form of imaging that does not use ionizing radiation. Ultrasound provides a safe, noninvasive method of measuring spinal canal diameter with great accuracy. It takes five minutes to perform. Thus it is ideally suited to preemployment screening. Based upon the assumption that a narrow spinal canal is a predisposing risk factor of back injury, ultrasound scans have found significant differences in spinal canal diameter in workers with and without low back pain. As was discussed briefly in the Epidemiology chapter, symptoms associated with disc degeneration or facet arthritis tend to be more disabling if the patient has a narrow canal. By definition, a stenotic condition increases the probability that a degenerative protrusion will compress the neural elements against the canal wall, since there is less space available for the nerve root(s) to pass around the protrusion without contact. In other words, those with wider spinal canals are better suited to tolerate spondylosis without back pain. These "wide-canal" patients have a greater safety factor built into their backs.

Consider the evidence from a three year study of 204 coal miners by Macdonald [33]. It was found that those men with the longest histories of low back pain and the longest periods of disability had significantly narrower canals, as measured by ultrasound. Of the days off work, 32% were lost by 22 miners with the narrowest 10% of spines. The widest canals occurred in those workers with no history of back pain, and the narrowest in those who had retired with a history of back pain. This finding suggests that ultrasonic spinal measurement could have important applications in the selection of heavy-industry workers. The authors conclude: "We believe that the specificity and sensitivity of any preemployment screening procedure for back pain would be improved by the combined use of spinal canal measurement and other parameters."

Strength Testing

Strength testing is based upon the concept that the exact nature of the physical tasks required of a worker dictates which physical attributes and abilities are important. Strength is a human attribute that can be quantitatively measured. It is associated with reduced propensity for injury. Therefore, it was proposed that some type of strength testing procedure which accurately simulated job performance would be valuable in matching job requirements to the physical capabilities of the employee. If a 1981 report from the National Institute for Occupational Safety and Health (NIOSH) is any indicator, strength testing is urgently needed to reduce the epidemic level of industrial injuries caused by overexertion [34]. The study found that overexertion was claimed as the cause of low back pain by over 60% of low back patients. Moreover, approximately 1 in 20 workers per year (500,000) experienced injuries related to overexertion, accounting for 25% of all reported occupational injuries in the United States. Some industries reported that over 50% of total reported injuries were caused by overexertion. Lastly, less than 33% of the patients with low back pain from overexertion ever returned to their previous job if they were disabled for a significant amount of time. The literature suggests that strength testing offers a viable solution to correcting the frequent mismatch between the physical demands of a job and the abilities of the worker.

Three types of tests are commonly used to measure a person's ability to exert lifting forces – isometric (static), isokinetic (dynamic), and isoinertial (psychophysical) tests. The majority of published research has focused on isometric strength testing.

Isometric testing is largely the creation of a research team led by Don Chaffin of the University of Michigan. It involves the exertion of a force in a given posture against a fixed resistance. The force is quantitatively measured and compared to the force requirements of the job. Accurate testing is highly dependent upon a detailed biomechanical job analysis that will isolate those job elements most responsible for high strength demands. Once these elements have been identified, it is possible to reconstruct the precise angle, height and magnitude of the primary work activity (be it lifting, pulling, reaching or pushing). Chaffin writes that "the technique measures the end result of a combination of processes having both physiological and psychological origins. As such it allows an objective scaling of what the person can and wants to physically do" [35]. Accordingly, the safety of isometric testing is great; no research to our knowledge has indicated major health hazards associated with testing, quite unlike the record of radiographic screening. The reliability of the test is also excellent, with a variation in multiple testing between 5% to10%. Additionally, the test equipment is low in cost, capable of simulating many different job requirements, and requires minimal time for administration.

If the extensive research of the Chaffin research team is any indication, isometric strength testing can predict the likelihood of future back problems. An example of the predictive capacity of the procedure was first reported by Chaffin in 1974 in an evaluation of 103 different jobs performed by 411 employees working in the electronics industry [35]. Three groups were formed, according to a job strength ratio which considered the job weight lifted and the strength of the employee. Those employees with a high strength capability were classified as an understressed group. Employees placed into jobs which more closely taxed their strength capability composed a considerably stressed group, while those employees unable to demonstrate as much isometric strength as required by their jobs were classified as overly stressed. Visits to the medical department were recorded over a one year period. Results indicated that the incidence of low back pain for the three stress groupings was significantly greater for those jobs populated by persons not demonstrating sufficient strength to equal or exceed the maximum predicted stress of their duties.

The same three group classifications were used in a later study to test the isometric condition of 551 people over the course of 18 months [36]. Over 900 manual handling jobs in six different plants were included in the study, each requiring a minimum 35-pound lift. Several tests were administered which simulated the lifting of a compact object close to the floor using a leg/squat lift technique, lifting a bulkier object from the floor using a back lift technique, and lifting an object from a table or bench using an arm lift. Results indicated that as the job strength requirement approached or exceeded the demonstrated isometric strength of workers on the job, the average back injury incidence and severity rates increased by 300%. Chaffin explains the vulnerability of the "overstressed" employee in this way: "When a person is performing an exertion close to his maximum strength, a sudden movement (ie slip) may cause tissue failure, be it muscular, ligamentous or disc related. Thus, occasional physical exertions of a heavy nature can be as damaging as more frequent exertions..."

Nearly identical results were observed in a biomechanical analysis of twenty jobs in a tire and rubber plant [37]. A comparison of the number of work injuries was made between employees hired on the basis of strength test performance and employees hired under the traditional medical criteria in effect at the plant. During the strength tests each applicant performed a five-second voluntary isometric exertion simulating arm and back lifting, as well as pushing and pulling. When all medical visits were considered, the back pain incidence rate for the 51 employees in the control group was observed to be over three times the incidence rate for those workers hired according to strength testing criteria.

A two-year analysis by Keyserling of 344 aluminum workers yielded similar findings [38]. Several different jobs were tested, including the most physically demanding tasks found anywhere in the plant. Each job was systematically broken down into strenuous task elements and the following variables were measured: type of task (ie push, pull, lift), the type of posture required (ie stand, sit, squat), required force needed to perform task, and the location of the hands in space. Using the same three group classification as noted in the prior two studies, it was determined that workers whose strength abilities were less than job requirements suffered higher injury rates than workers whose strength matched or exceeded job demands. Significant relationships were found among worker strength, job demands, and medical incidents on four of nine tests, with the "weak" group experiencing between 1.25 to 2.71 times the injury rates suffered by the matched and "strong" groups. Similar trends were observed in the remainder of the data. Interestingly enough, excess strength was not found to be of protective value in the prevention of medical problems. No differences in injury rates were observed between workers whose strengths matched job demands and workers whose strengths exceeded job demands.

While these studies clearly indicate the efficacy of isometric testing, the procedure is not beyond criticism. Because isometric lifting is a static test, the procedure traditionally test only in one geometric plane of movement, as opposed to normal human function which usually cuts across three planes. Furthermore, static lifting tests strength in only one position devoid of joint movement. It does not allow dynamic changes in posture, joint loading, and muscle length/tension ratios. Lastly, it does not account for acceleration and deceleration of body segments, which make up 82% to 84% of body movements.

Dynamic strength testing resolves most of the disadvantages outlined above. As an alternative to isometric testing, isokinetic lifting represents a better simulation of the actual lifting task by allowing measurement of forces through the entire range of motion. This can give dynamic testing the distinct advantage of identifying those who intentionally put out submaximal effort at various points in the arc of motion, a valuable tool in isolating the low back malingerer. Although isokinetic testing may identify consistent pathologic patterns among back-injured individuals and is also safe and reliable, the equipment cost is beyond the budget of the average industrial company. The other disadvantage is that the equipment does not easily accommodate lifting movements out of the sagittal plane.

Yet another type of strength test is psychophysical analysis. These tests are similar to dynamic tests in that the individual is required to perform a simulated job task, but is permitted to adjust the amount of task load by increasing or decreasing the weight from an arbitrary starting point unknown to the subject. Simulating the frequency and repetition of work acitivity, several lifts are performed with the load being readjusted to a tolerable level. The weight level selected by the subject as most comfortable and safe is considered the safe upper limit for that individual. According to Chaffin et al. this method "may be the most accurate method of determining a person's acceptable performance limit for a given task" [39]. Troup argues that psychophysical tests of acceptable load (isokinetic) and acceptable isometric force are as sensitive to the prevalence of back pain as maximal isometric strength tests. Such tests are also safer and cheaper to administer than isokinetic strength tests [40].

Griffin et al. evaluated the differences in psychophysical lifting capability between 335 subjects with and without low back pain [41]. The participants were requested to select the maximal weight that was thought to be comfortable for lifting from floor to table at five-minute intervals throughout a working day. It was found that subjects with previous back pain chose acceptable loads that were on average 4.1 kg (9 lbs) for men and 2.2 kg (5 lbs) for women less than those without previous back pain. The results do not indicate whether the procedure can actually predict the future incidence or severity of back pain, something an effective screening test must be able to distinguish. Troup did explore the predictive power of psychophysical analysis in a group of 1,741 men and 1,150 women that were given a variety of acceptable lifting exercises [40]. Followed up one year later, the test battery predicted back pain in only 35% of the male and 37% of the female participants. Thus, none of the tests were of any value in predicting new cases of low back pain. In fact, this method of strength testing was no more accurate in predicting low back pain than a combination of tests based on respiratory function, administered to all subjects.

Job Rating Programs

Yet another method of worker selection is a job rating program. Similar to strength testing, job rating programs are structured attempts to evaluate the job as well as the worker, thereby obtaining an ideal match between the two. The central characteristic of job rating emphasizes ability, rather than disability. Consequently, many handicapped, older workers, and workers previously rejected by general health screening tests are able to be integrated into positions custom tailored to their physical strengths. With an emphasis on identifying suitable work for people of varying abilities, job ratings were first utilized by the armed forces during World War II to distribute the millions of new recruits to positions with clear-cut physical qualifications.

Hanman is credited with introducing the military to a program known as PULHES [42]. The evaluation of the individual had six parts, corresponding to each letter of the program name: P - physical capacity or stamina, U - upper extremity, L - lower extremity, H - hearing, E - eyesight, S - neuropsychiatric. Each factor was numerically graded by an industrial physician and compared to a description of job requirements as evaluated by a job analyst. Lastly, a placement officer selected the job best suited to the workers skills and physical abilities. Because Hanman was selecting the job for the worker (and not vice versa), the program can be most accurately classified as a "pre-placement examination", rather than a "pre-employment examination." The program was so successful that it inspired the Canadian and British armies to adopt a similar rating system with slight modification. One of the most current job rating systems in use, the Medical Standards Project of San Bernardino County (CA) further refined Hanman's original list of physical components thought to influence human performance capabilities. Fleishman found nine abilities (rated on a one to seven scale) necessary for evaluating the physical requirements of work tasks: dynamic strength, trunk strength, static strength, explosive strength, extension flexibility, dynamic flexibility, gross body coordination, gross body equilibrium, and stamina [43].

As far as the efficacy of job ratings, Snook concludes: "It is not surprising that so much time and effort has gone into the development of job rating programs. The programs appear to provide valuable information regarding worker capabilities and job requirements. It is surprising, however, that not a single study could be found that objectively evaluated the effectiveness of any of the job rating programs in reducing the incidence, severity or cost of musculoskeletal injuries in the workplace. These programs have good potential, but they remain unproven with respect to injury reduction" [44].

Job Design (Ergonomics)

Ergonomics is the study of people in relation to their working environment, integrating concepts and theoretical knowledge from the scientific disciplines of occupational biomechanics, anatomy, physiology and engineering. Whereas pre-employment screening is concerned with selecting appropriate workers for duties with varying physical requirements, the objective of ergonomics is the opposite -- designing (and redesigning) the job to fit the capabilities and limitations of the worker. A basic ergonomic principle is that the work load should be minimized or distributed in an optimal manner. Effective job design seeks to reduce the health hazards of activities and postures related to industrial low back pain. By limiting low back strain and stress caused by manual handling (especially excessive lifting), prolonged sitting and vibration, work injuries can be reduced. In this way, ergonomics serves as a method of primary prevention, a first line of defense against back attack.

Adequate workplace design is mandatory when one considers that lifting, sitting, and vibration, discussed at length in the Epidemiology chapter, are responsible for the much of low back injury. Snook [10] and others have found that more than half of all compensable back incidents have been related to manual handling, with lifting implicated in 37% to 49% of all cases; pushing, 9% to 16%; pulling, 6% to 9%; and carrying, 5% to 8% [10]. According to Snook, approximately 70% of worksite back injuries are caused by lifting that is below knuckle height (below 31 inches), a significant finding considering that low lifting composes two-thirds of all industrial lifts. Furthermore, twisting body movement has been related to 9% to 18% of back cases, bending to 12% to 14% of back injury, and slips or falls 7% to 13% of low back problems.

Biomechanical evaluation of the postural demands of work activity is central to ergonomic prevention of low back pain. Once the most stressful physical requirements of a specific work activity are isolated as individual components, alternatives can be suggested by the ergonomist or occupational health specialist which will alter the working methods of employees in a manner that reduces musculoskeletal fatigue. The literature demonstrates conclusively that work activity slightly modified to help the individual distribute the load more uniformly can make all the difference in preserving the health of the employee. Those involved with manual handling are most vulnerable to back injury, therefore it is this group that has the most to gain from ergonomic modification of the workplace.

Lifting Techniques

Industry has developed a wide variety of mechanical aids to assist with heavy weights and forces associated with materials handling, including hand trucks, carts, hoists, conveyors and cranes. Theoretically, these aids should reduce stressful postures, but in many settings these devices are ignored by workers because they are not efficiently integrated into the work environment. The employee that chooses to manually roll a hundred pound barrel instead of using a hand cart which might take substantially more time to load is going to frustrate attempts to reduce back injury. Likewise, a nurse cannot be expected to use a hoist to lift patients under emergency conditions if the device requires complex maneuvering of the patient, bed or other objects. Indeed, no hospital exists with hoists alongside every bed. It is not the introduction of ergonomic aids that will produce beneficial results, but the compliance of the workforce in using tools that do not hinder their productivity or sacrifice performance. In other words, the ergonomic device must be practically suited to the requirements of the job. It would appear that an aid will not be completely accepted by the workforce unless the ergonomic procedure is no more time-consuming than the time needed to execute the activity manually.

Several findings provide compelling evidence illustrating the physiological costs (both short and long term) of poor manual handling techniques. For instance, Snook has demonstrated that the pressure generated upon the intravertebral disc is 33% greater when the arms are outstretched than when the object is lifted from the floor but kept close to the body [10]. Similarly, a 20% forward lean will result in an increase of energy output by 30% to 50%, leading to increased fatigue and injuries. One example of this phenomenon dates back to 1963 when Scholz et al. showed that the avoidance of working in a stooped posture reduced the calories consumed per shift by an average of 25% and that the heart rate slowed by about 20% [45]. Fatigue reduction was also observed by Andersson et al. in an analysis of seat design [46]. They found that a backward inclination to the seat produced less strain and effort to the paraspinal muscles. Such a finding has tremendous application to the millions of office workers and drivers confined to long periods of sitting, the position that causes the greatest intradiscal pressure by far. The operative principle in this case is that when the proportion of mechanical energy that goes into static effort (bent back, prolonged sitting) is increased, the efficiency of the performed work task is decreased. Another factor relevant to ergonomic evaluation is the speed of lifting, which causes a 15% to 20% increase in power demand if the object is lifted rapidly. The symmetry of the lift is yet another factor to consider. Asymmetrical lifting is more often the rule than the exception in industry. Symmetrical lifting is defined as lifting in the sagittal plane only with the lift centered in front of a person, whereas asymmetrical lifting takes place on two planes, turning the body while continuing to lift.

One study which examined the effects of symmetrical and asymmetrical lifting on the body, as well as several other risk factors, is by Mital et al.[47]. The study was designed to investigate the effects of lifting height, lifting frequency, box size, and symmetrical and asymmetrical containers (dependent on the location of the load center of gravity) on the maximum acceptable symmetrical/asymmetrical weight of lift, resulting heart rate, and oxygen uptake. Eighteen healthy adult males perfomed 60 different lifting activities involving two lifting heights, three lifting frequencies, and five containers.

The degree of symmetry of both the lifting style and load characteristics had a definite impact on lifting capability. Symmetrical lifting technique allowed the subjects to work with 8.44% more weight than an asymmetrical lifting style, yet there was no difference in heart rate and very little difference in oxygen uptake between the two methods. The maximum acceptable weight of lift decreased in direct proportion with the box dimensions. When the box increased from 30 to 48 cm to 45 to 72 cm, the maximum lift weight decreased by approximately 5%, and the largest box size (60 to 96 cm) led to a further decrease of 5%. Height also influenced lifting, as 8.54% more weight was lifted from the floor to 81 cm height than from 81 to 152 cm height. Furthermore, 7% less weight was lifted when the lift frequency increased from one to four lifts per minute, and an additional decrease of 8.5% was observed when frequency increased from four to eight lifts per minute. Both height and frequency substantially influenced heart rate and oxygen uptake values. The cumulative results of the study found that 21.3% more symmetrical weight was lifted using a symmetrical method when compared to an asymmetrical object lifted asymmetrically. Lifting capacity is most likely reduced because of greater intra-abdominal pressure and higher spinal shear stresses which are associated with asymmetrical lifting.

As the reader might have guessed, a great deal of ergonomic research is focused on lifting, studied in terms of proper technique and ideal weight guidelines. Since lifting technique is more directly related to low back education and training, that preventive approach will be discussed in the last section of this chapter. Several methods have been proposed to help determine excessive loads predisposing to low back pain, including the lifting-strength rating, job severity index, psychophysical tables, and guidelines from the National Institute for Occupational Safety and Health. One detailed example is a psychophysical strength index constructed by Snook, based upon the percentage of the working population that can be expected to perform a certain task without overexertion [10]. The study evaluated 191 compensable back claimants and found that proper design of manual handling tasks could reduce the incidence of back pain by up to one-third.

According to the index, a task was considered relatively safe if 75% or more of the working population could handle it without overexertion. Those tasks that less than 75% of the working population could complete without overexertion were three times as likely to expose workers to low back injury. As an example of a recommended weight value, the author calculated from the data that 75% of industrial male workers can lift a 45 pound common size tote box from the floor, or exert a 69 pound initial horizontal pushing force without overexertion. Snook argues that while the majority of all manual handling jobs (66%) involve tasks that 75% of the working population can comfortably perform, it is clear that the remaining occupations are exposing employees to increased risk. Similarly, both Chaffin [35,36] and Keyserling [37,38] have found a threefold increase in the risk of back injury when the job requirements exceeded the strength capacity of the worker. Such industries should be especially conscious to the dangers of back pain, and would be well advised to adopt every ergonomic guideline that is available, feasible and affordable.

Workplace Design

In the office setting, unnecessary bending, twisting, reaching and prolonged sitting can be reduced by adjusting the height of tables and chairs to an optimum level. A low table may cause kyphosis of the lumbar spine, increasing the load on the vertebra. On the other hand, a high table can cause abduction of the arms and elevation of the shoulders as neck strain, causing fatigue in the shoulder and cervical muscles. The application of ergonomic principles to the chair emphasizes ideal thigh support, lumbar support at the level of the fourth and fifth vertebrae, inclination of the backrest to an angle between 100 and 110 degrees, and a seat design that permits the feet to rest firmly on the floor or foot support. Armrests are also important in reducing pressure on the seat surface, load on the spine, and facilitating rising from the chair.

An industrial environment designed according to ergonomic principles would be structured in accordance with the fundamental objective of minimizing the distance between the worker and the center of mass of the object being manipulated (lift, push, pull, rotate, reach etc. . . .). Obstructions over which a worker must lean to manipulate an object must be eliminated. Chaffin provides the following examples of ergonomic mechanical aids [48]:

1. Roller conveyors which allow objects to be pulled in toward the body before lifting or powered conveyors to bring containers to the worker.
2. Gravity-fed slides (or shelves) which present items to the worker.
3. Machine designs which have the workpiece or part being manufactured located close to the operator.
4. Tilting of large stock bins to present parts closer to the operator.
5. Enough room for a worker to walk around large bins or pallets of parts to avoid having to reach and lean forward to remove parts from the opposite sides.

Ergonomics and Vibration

Vehicular vibration associated with driving is another risk factor that affects the majority of inhabitants in modern industrial society. Epidemiological studies have shown that vibration can be particularly hazardous to the seated spine where the spine's natural frequency is resonated in the critical 4 to 6 Hz range, corresponding to the vehicles own oscillations. Vibration within this range will cause the spine to resonate, leading to fatigue and failure of the paraspinal muscles and a decrease in load-bearing capability. The morbidity caused by vibration is magnified by the postural and muscular components of sitting stress. Consequently, professional drivers (bus, taxi, or truck) who drive over half the work day may be risking premature disc degeneration and back pain through long-term exposure to vibration. The risk of low back pain and herniated disc is two to four times greater for these occupations than the general public. Even the average commuter traveling over 20 miles a day has a risk two to four times greater than the public. What can be done to help diminish the effects of this industrial phenomenon?

Modification of the seat is the focal point of ergonomic research to better insulate the driver from road shock while providing improved lumbar and thigh support. As Troup attests, "the design of the seat is, therefore, the most valuable single item in preventing back symptoms in drivers" [49]. Conventional car seats tend to be too upright, causing measurable spinal stress as the head and shoulders are forced to bend forward, inducing a flexor torque that is only made worse by vibration. The design of a seat with a back rest inclination of 110 degrees or more and a seat inclination of 6 degrees was developed by Anderssson et al. in response to such problems [46]. Using the model seat, spinal stress was reduced by better load distribution over the back rest as well as the seat. Muscular stress can be further diminished if the vertical height of the seat above the floor is set as high as possible without causing undue pressure on the back of the thighs.

In addition to proper angulation, the ideal seat should utilize firm cushions instead of the soft seat cushions that allow vibration in the 4 to 8 Hz range. Vibration can be further reduced with a seat suspension system. Most professional truck drivers have adopted these seat design guidelines for their own vehicles, but automobiles for the general public (nearly a billion vehicles worldwide) have with few exceptions failed to implement these ergonomic principles. Modification of the driver seat by the world's leading automobile manufacturers could have a dramatic influence in preserving the health of the low back and limiting the incidence of future back pain.

Empirical Evidence

Attempts at reducing the incidence of back pain through the use of mechanical aids and proper work station design have been inconsistent. Benson published one of the few articles to document the benefits of ergonomics in a review of six industries that adopted ergonomic task redesign and achieved a reduction in the incidence and cost of compensable back pain [50]. A 33% reduction in long-term sick leave related to musculoskeletal illness was observed by

Westgaard et al. following the implementation of ergonomic improvements [51]. A significant impediment to discussing the track record of ergonomics is the paucity of long-term research, not to mention the problem of isolating the effects of ergonomics from the confounding influences of other preventive variables constantly introduced into the work place. Disagreement between epidemiological and ergonomic research is another source of confusion. Argument over the industrial (or individual) source of back pain has led to a great variety of recommended ergonomic guidelines for every imaginable risk factor.

An extensive review of both epidemiological and ergonomic research by Dul et al. [52] detailed the divergence of opinion between the two fields. The study was based on sixteen ergonomic and epidemiological text books published after 1975, including material by Chaffin et al.[39]. Significant differences among the ergonomic recommendations to help resolve risk factors were noted. For instance, three ergonomic texts suggested that the classical lifting technique (straight back, bent knees) is most appropriate, while four other texts suggested that the load should be lifted as close to body as possible. Calculated maximum lifting weight is another controversial guideline, with a recommended range of 27 to 80 kg (60 to 176 lbs) for men and 10 to 64 kg (22 to 141 lbs) for women! The great diversity in weight levels suggest that criteria other than back pain have played a role in the calculations, such as factors related to energy consumption or perceived exertion. Half of these ergonomic texts do not indicate the criteria or references on which these numbers are based, prompting the author to state ". . . in principle, most guidelines are not formulated specifically for prevention of low back pain". Dul notes that even in cases where the references are provided, "it turns out that only a few guidelines are based upon a single back load criterion such as EMG of back muscles, biomechanical compression forces on L5-S1, intra-discal pressure, or intra-abdominal pressure."

In addition to disagreement within the ergonomic literature over work techniques, there is marked disagreement between ergonomics and epidemiology when it comes to recognition of individual risk factors. The ergonomic review indicated that about 40% of the concrete guidelines did not even include individual risk factors. A comparison of the leading individual risk factors revealed that ergonomic guidelines did not correspond with the risk factors recognized by the epidemiological studies. For instance, 20% of all ergonomic guidelines included sex as an individual risk factor, while the epidemiological studies did not even consider it among the top six risk factors. Considering the utter lack of consensus in this area, Dul states: "This means that in principle ergonomic guidelines are not specific enough for the protection of certain groups of workers with reduced capacity such as elderly workers, workers who had a period of low back pain before, and so on." From this comprehensive review one can conclude that ergonomic research must be specifically directed at the prevention of low back pain to provide more reliable and valid guidelines.

Education and Training

Education and training is the third major component of back pain prevention. Traditionally directed toward workers, education in safe lifting technique and physical fitness training are the most commonly used prevention programs in industry. As was mentioned earlier, safe lifting techniques have received the most attention, in an attempt to cut down on the 50% of all compensable back pain incidents associated with manual lifting tasks. Since the articles by Brackett in 1924 which first identified the possible dangers of lifting a heavy load from the ground with the back in the fully flexed position, ergonomists have sought to identify safer lifting techniques and load limits.

Lifting Techniques

Two primary lifting techniques have been proposed as least stressful to the biomechanics of the spine. The "classical" method emphasizes a straight back and bent knees while lifting with the leg muscles. The key to the method is on pivoting with the pelvis -- and not at the critical lumbosacral junction. Anderson and Chaffin proved that this lifting technique yielded lower L5-S1 disc compression, low back ligament strain and strength requirements than lifting with a bent back and "locked" knees [53]. However, this finding was disputed by Garg et al. in a report that could not confirm a clear biomechanical rationale for using the "classical" method [54]. Brown agrees with this assessment in his book on manual handling: "there is clear evidence... that there has not been any significant reduction in injuries due to lifting and handling, etc., over the past 30 years when the straight back, bent knees lifting method has been advocated" [55]. (Figure 5-1)

The second significant lifting technique refined the mechanics of the initial technique by recommending that objects should be lifted as close the body as possible. This latter technique was thought to be an improvement of the "classical" method because it recognized that in many instances the load is too large to be lifted between the legs. In order for the load to pass the knees, the distance between the load and body becomes relatively large, in effect increasing the lever arm of the lift and resulting in additional stress on the spine. It is also argued that the "classical" method requires an asymmetrical position of the feet and correspondingly of the trunk to preserve a balanced posture, another source of spinal stress. More recently, other principles have been incorporated within these techniques, such as smooth lifting without jerking, turning with the feet instead of twisting the trunk (reducing axial torque), and correct positioning of the feet, chin, arms and hands.

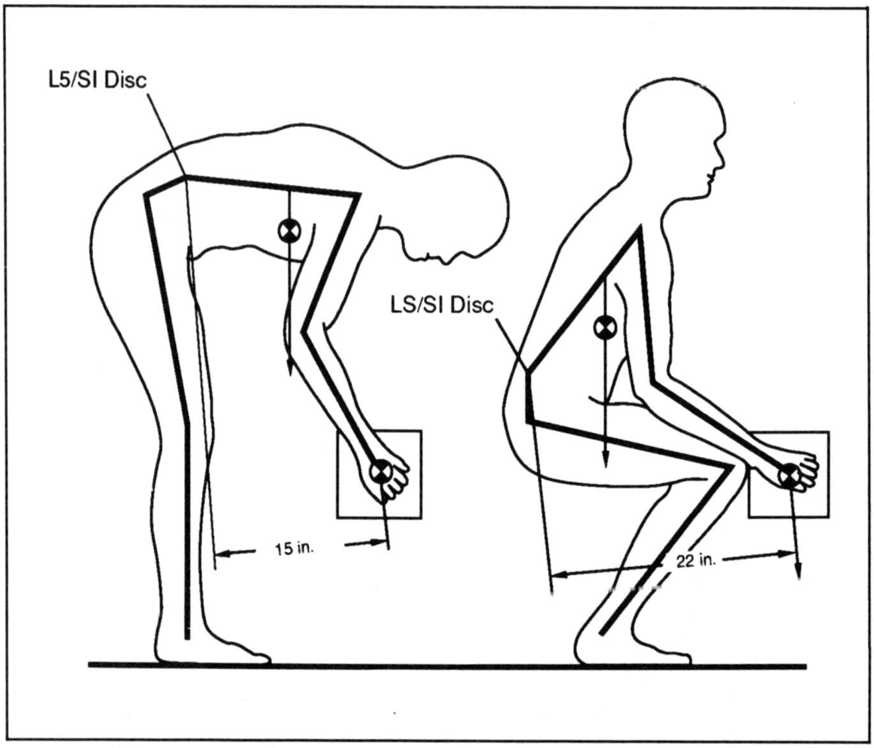

Fig 5-1: This figure illustrates that "correct" lifting techniques may not always reduce disc stress. If a worker lifts a bulky object that cannot fit between the knees, the larger lever arm to the L5-S1 disc will result in greater torque at that level than stooped lifting. (Modified from Chafin, D. B. and Anderson, G.: Occupational Biomechanics: John Wiley and Sons, 1984)

While the theories underlying the use of safer lifting techniques are logical, empirical evidence supporting these methods is not convincing. Relatively few studies have reported significant reduction in back disability as a result of these methods; nearly all reports are uncontrolled and short term. The National Institute for Occupational Safety and Health (NIOSH) has concluded that the value of safe lifting is open to question because of the non-existence of a controlled study demonstrating a consequent drop in manual handling accident rate or back injury [56]. Two such studies by Glover [57] and Miller [58] reported a 65% and 70% disability reduction. Several studies have reported little or no effect in back pain incidence after implementing safe lifting principles [59]. According to a study of 191 compensable back cases, Snook concluded that just as many injuries were experienced by employers who provided safe lifting training as by employers who did not provide training [10]. In fact, data from this report found that those companies with training programs sustained roughly 20% more injuries than companies without any training (not statistically significant). It should be noted that training was provided more often by the larger employer and the employer with the greatest exposure to manual handling injury. Unfortunately, this study made no attempt to evaluate the quality of the training procedures.

Physical Fitness Training

One reason that many training programs have failed to reduce the incidence and/or severity of back-related disability is because employers and employees have both neglected the importance of proper physical conditioning. The argument is often made that the muscular stress of work often is equal to or greater than the muscular stress of athletics. Yet unlike the athlete who understands the need to match cardiovascular or muscular fitness with the exact physical requirements of the activity, millions of workers do not recognize the magnitude or consequences of the mismatch until back pain strikes them down. Granted, it is utterly impractical to have employees work out on weight machines or run a few miles before the start of the workday, but a brief exercise period that stimulates blood flow and enhances flexibility is reasonable. It seems ironic that the athlete will never participate in strenuous activity without stretching beforehand, while the average worker (or manager) has never even considered stretching as a prerequisite to job activity. While the application of these basic principles is observed in every sport as a primary means of injury prevention, the similarities between the athlete and the industrial or corporate employee have not been recognized by most companies. Unfortunately, the connection between sports and work has not yet been made, despite the fact that up to 90% of back injuries are caused by muscle insufficiency — weak, tight, fatigued, tense, previously injured, or cold muscles [60].

Numerous articles have been published indicating the value of physical fitness in reducing back injury. As was clearly demonstrated in the epidemiology chapter, the four year study by Cady monitoring exercise and injury among 1652 firefighters is probably the single best example of the need to improve the fitness of any workforce [61]. The firemen were organized into three fitness groups according to five cardiovascular criteria. The measurements included heart rate and diastolic blood pressure after exercise, spine flexibility measurements, total isometric strength of selected muscle groups, and endurance work measured at the end of twenty minutes of heart-rate-controlled exercise. Cady found that approximately 7% of the least fit group experienced low back pain, compared to 3% of the middle fitness group and less than 1% for the most fit group. A subsequent follow-up study reported that the introduction of cardiovascular fitness programs improved stamina, endurance, strength and flexibility [62]. As a result of increased cardiovascular fitness, even without significant increases in strength and flexibility, workers' compensation costs were reduced 25%.

The reason that the most physically fit firefighters experienced such a low incidence of back pain is not difficult to explain. Proper lifting mechanics are substituted for increasingly hazardous mechanics as fatigue sets in during job performance. Those individuals performing repetitive manual labor are especially at risk. A worker who would earlier pick up an object by flexing at the knees and hips and keeping the spine erect begins to lift by flexing the spine and flexing less at the knees and hips. This occurs because the center of gravity, located approximately at the level of the pelvis, moves much less when just the spine is flexed than when the knees and hips are flexed. As a result, more energy is expended lifting an object properly because one must lift not only the object but also one's center of gravity [63]. Logically, the better conditioned workers would be able to maintain proper postural mechanics longer than lesser conditioned workers.

Another point to consider is that physical fatigue is often accompanied by mental fatigue, leading to a reduction in work efficiency and accuracy. Poor concentration leads to accidents involving not only the back but other parts of the body. Additionally, the positive effects of regular exercise programs could be transferred from the workplace to the home, as employees take a more active role in caring for their bodies. Such programs can inspire one to stop smoking and improve the diet. Since smoking and obesity have been implicated as risk factors increasing the probability of back pain incidence, elimination of these factors may help reduce the frequency of this condition [63].

While all employees would benefit from physical conditioning, the methods used to improve the health of the workforce is practically limited by available space, time, and cost constraints. Implementation of a brief warm-up exercise period before or during the workday could be the ideal solution in preventing future back injury. Stretching is considered by Locke to be the most fundamental aspect of fitness development and maintenance because it improves flexibility, allowing the muscle to be stretched further in a strain-producing situation without being injured [60]. Furthermore, stretching "reduces muscle tension, improves coordination, increases the range of motion of joints, enhances circulation, develops body awareness and helps provide a sense of personal well-being." Flexibility exercises offers other advantages as well: they can be done in any location and at any time, and are simple enough that most employees are able to do all the stretches. The exercises do not require special clothing or equipment, nor do they require much space. In its simplest stage, the cost of implementing a stretching routine would not require a large capital outlay. Similarly, an uncomplicated program would be more attractive to the workforce, encouraging participation and compliance.

Comprehensive Back Education & Training Programs

Although the instruction of safe lifting techniques or stretching exercises in and of themselves has not made much of an impact in reducing worker disability, the integration of ideal lifting methods with a more comprehensive back education program has been significantly more successful. Emphasizing the same subjects and training strategies used in low back schools, many companies have transformed such programs from a form of treatment to a form of prevention. No longer willing to continue with a "laissez-faire" approach to back disability, many companies are actively discussing the issues of industrial low back pain in the context of anatomy, physiology, body mechanics, posture and physical fitness. The objective is to develop the employee's awareness of back disability through education in an effort to persuade and motivate the worker to adopt work habits based upon intelligence and a cautious respect for the potential hazards of even the simplest work activities.

Unfortunately, it is not enough to merely present to the workforce the facts, figures and recommendations associated with back problems. Prevention programs that do not implement a focused strategy that encourages the direct participation of the employee are doomed to failure. According to Morris, the ability to motivate compliance is the single most important component of a prevention program [64]. How can this elusive factor be achieved? Morris suggests several variables essential to success. To begin with, a Recognition phase is proposed as the starting point, demonstrating to the employees the existence of a problem and their role and involvement in it. Second, the employees are provided with a basic understanding of the etiology and natural history of lumbar back pain, considered the Knowledge phase. This phase is instrumental in the validation of reasons for behavior change. The Relevance phase develops a personal involvement of the employee as an appreciation of the previously thoughtless use of stressful movements is addressed. An Alteration phase teaches the worker how to change his work behavior by using techniques for reducing spinal stress caused by improper lifting or posture. The fifth phase demonstrates application of the principles of proper back care, taking the employees through an exercise of lifting, bending, carrying and reaching consistent with their job requirements. This phase is known as the Practical phase, helping the employee to develop a body awareness of the correct low stress postures and body mechanics. The last phase is aggressive implementation and follow-up, utilizing specially trained employee "trainers" and supportive attitudes from management to maintain and evaluate the efficacy of the program. (Figure 5-2)

Morris offers several examples of how a well-planned, comprehensive prevention program can reduce costs associated with low back injuries. Lockheed Missile and Space Company experienced a 68% reduction in their annual average total back injury costs over a 14 month period after implementation of a back injury prevention program at their Sunnyvale, CA location [65]. Even greater gains were realized by the American Biltrite-Chelsea plant, where a program emphasizing employee education and in-house conservative therapy resulted in a 90% decrease in worker's compensation costs [66]. At Capital Wire

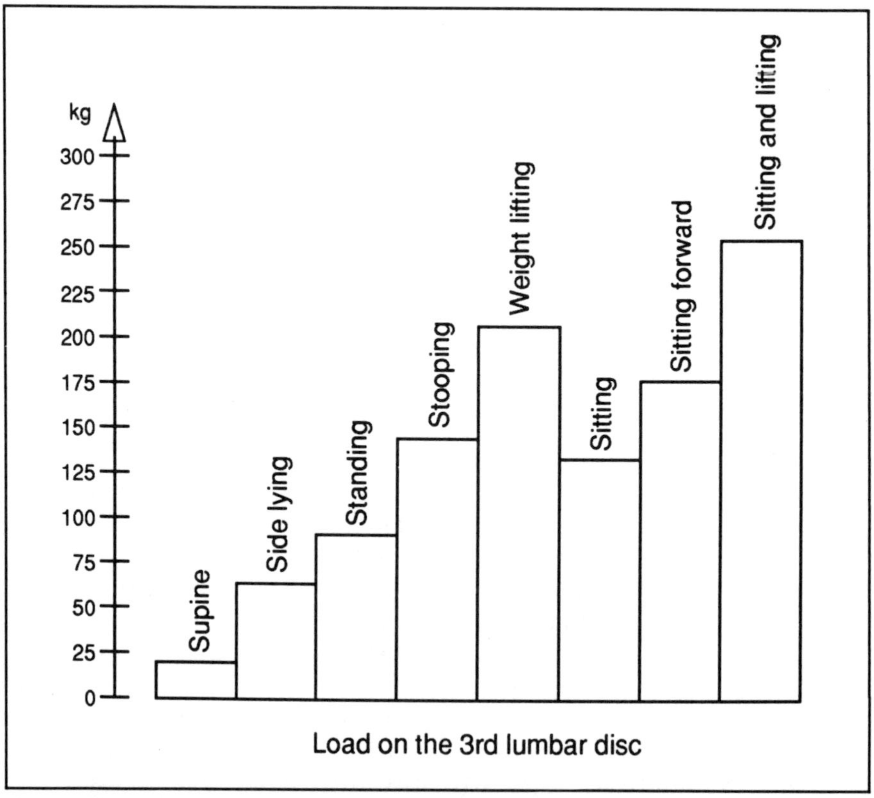

Fig 5-2: This graph shows the tremendous variation in stress on the L3 disc when the body assumes different positions (modified from Nachemson, A: In vivo discometry in the lumbar discs with irregular nucleograms. Acta Orthop. Scand. 36:426, 1965.)

and Cable Company, the total cost of low back injuries was reduced from $191,549 over two years before the prevention program to just under $7,000 over 20 months after implementation [64]. Back injury illness was reduced 95% at a Burlington factory after a program was instituted, incorporating individual counseling, back exercises and instruction on how to perform various job function without causing spinal stress [67]. Among the 300 employees, one third experienced more than 400 days of absenteeism due to back problems, yet the same employees missed only 19 days of work a year after the program initiation. Other uncontrolled studies have reported similar findings for preventive type back schools. Two years after the adoption of a program modeled after the California Back School, the Southern Pacific Company achieved a 22% reduction in the number of low back cases and a 43% reduction in lost work days among a group of 30,000 employees [68]. Johnson reported a 70% and 90% reduction in the number of injuries and cost of injuries using the Atlanta Back School after two years at PPG industries [69].

Management, Labor, and Medical Practitioner Training

Prevention of low back injury does not stop with the education and training of the workforce. Snook argues that reducing the economic and anatomic costs of low back injury will not be maximized until it is recognized that employees are merely one group in a system which tends to promote disability by encouraging labor-management confrontation and discouraging return to work of the injured employee [70]. Doctors who down play injuries in hopes of returning a patient back to work do not help the problem either. In short, training programs must be extended to include management, labor unions and medical practitioners. These three groups have a substantial role to play in disability reduction; unless plans are made to change their perception of back pain, the attitudes and practices of the corporate, legal and medical establishment is going to limit the success of company training programs to the most superficial results.

A more enlightened prevention strategy will aid management in establishing a positive acceptance of back pain, instead of an adversarial approach automatically doubting the validity of the injury before further information becomes available. Communication between the worker and management is critical, as a company that turns a deaf ear on the employee's situation creates and reinforces the worker's desire to correct the perceived injustice through litigation. Under this scenario, malingering is initiated and consequently rewarded. Management can also be faulted for perpetuating disability because many companies will not allow the return of the employee unless he is 100% healthy. Rigid union rules prohibiting early return to work share in the blame, many believing that the worker is entitled to time off for even a minor injury.

Although a seemingly pragmatic decision, research by McGill [71] and Rosen [72] has shown that the longer a disabled worker is off work, the less chance that individual has of ever returning to work. Their data, accepted by most occupational medicine scholars, indicates that workers who are off more than six months have only a 50% possibility of ever returning to productive employment. After one year, the probability drops to 25%, and an abscence of two years makes the chances of return to work almost zero. Furthermore, the transformation of an acute injury to a chronic condition increases the likelihood of illness behavior, a condition whereby the psychological aspects of pain become more significant than pain produced by the actual injury. Snook suggests the importance of providing alternative part-time work specifically modified to the diminished abilities of the injured worker as a means of hastening the return of the worker. "Effective management will do everything possible to encourage the worker to return, because there is only a limited amount of time before losing control of the disability."

Summary

Prevention of back pain and disability should begin at the individual level. Placing an employee in a job suited to his/her strengths and physical talents seems an appropriate place to start. Strength testing and pre-placement physical examinations can help insure that each employee is given the job that best fits his/her capabilities. For those workers who have already invested much time and effort in jobs inimical to their back health, proper design of tools, seats, desks, and work areas would hold some promise for extending their careers.

It appears that the total health of the individual cannot be separated from his/her health at work. Work programs which teach employees how to care for their backs and how to remain physically fit should pay great dividends in lowered injury rates and fewer missed days from work. Creating a caring, non-confrontational environment between employers and their workforce would considerably reduce overtreatment, legal expenses, and other inefficiency that are driving up the costs of low back pain.

References

1. Snook SH: Low back pain in industry. In White AA, Gordon SL (eds.): Symposium on Idiopathic Low Back Pain. St. Louis, CV Mosby, 1982, p 23.
2. Spengler DM, Bigos SJ, Martin NA, et al: Back injuries in industry: A retrospective study. I. Overview and cost analysis. Spine 11:241, 1986.
3. Dwyer AP: Backache and its prevention. Clin Orthop 222:35-43, 1987.
4. Cain C: Big employers increasing health cost control study. Business Insurance. March 31, 1983.
5. American Medical Association Council on Occupational Health: Guiding principles of medical examinations in industry. JAMA 161:975-978, 1956.
6. Lloyd DCEF, JDG Troup: Recurrent back pain and its prediction. J Soc Occup Med 33:66-74, 1983.
7. Dillane JB, Fry J, Kalton G: Acute back symptoms - a study from general practice. Br Med Journ 2:82-84, 1966.
8. Rowe ML: Backache at Work. Fairport, NY. Perinton Press, 1983.
9. Chaffin DB, Herrin GD, Keyserling WM: Pre-employment strength testing in selecting workers for materials handling jobs. US Dept Health Educ Welfare (NIOSH) CDC-99-74-62, 1976.
10. Snook SH, Campanelli RA, Hart JW: A study of three preventive approaches to low back injury. J Occup Med 20:478, 1978.
11. Rowe ML: Low back pain in industry. J Occup Med 11:161-169, 1964.
12. Rowe ML: Low back pain in industry. J Occup Med 13:476-478, 1971.
13. Nachemson A: The lumbar spine. An orthopedic challenge. Spine 1:59, 1976.

14. Scavone JG, Latshaw RF, Ropler GW: Use of lumbar spine films. Statistical evaluation at a university teaching school. JAMA 246:1105, 1981.
15. Friedman MM, Fischer FJ, VanDemark RE: Lumbosacral roentgenograms of 100 soldiers. Amer J Roentgenol 55:292, 1946.
16. Ford LT: from article by Edeiken J, Karasick D: Use of radiography for screening employees for risk of low back disability. J of Occup Med 28(10):995-997, 1986.
17. Splithoff CA: Lumbosacral junction; roentgenographic comparison of patients with and without backaches. J Amer Med Assoc 152:1610, 1953.
18. Fullenlove TM, Williams AJ: Comparative roentgen findings in symptomatic and asymptomatic backs. Radiology 63:572, 1957.
19. Stewart SF: Pre-employment examination of the back. J Bone Joint Surg 29:215, 1947.
20. Marsh HO, Robold C: A practical solution for the industrial back problem including x-ray examination. Compensation Med 4:21, 1952.
21. McGill CM: Industrial back problems; a control program. J Occup Med 10:174, 1968.
22. Runge CF: Pre-existing structural defects and severity of compensation back injuries. Indust Med Surg 27:249, 1958.
23. Kosiak M, Aurelius JR, Hartfiel WF: The low back problem - an evaluation. J Occup Med 10:588, 1968.
24. Connell MA: Bony anomalies of the low back in relation to back injury. South Med J 61:482-486, 1968.
25. Leggo C, Mathiasen H: Preliminary results of a pre-employment back x-ray program for state traffic control officers. J of Occup Med 15(12):973-974, 1973.
26. Montgomery CH: Preemployment back x-rays. J of Occup Med 18(7):495-498, 1976.
27. Injury experience of reporters to the National Safety Council, 1926 to 1973. Accident facts, 1974.
28. Redfield JT: The low back x-ray as a pre-employment screening tool in the forest products industry. J of Occup Med 13(5):219-226, 1971.
29. Gibson ES, Martin RH, Terry CW: Incidence of low back pain and preplacement x-ray screening. J Occup Med 8:515, 1980.
30. Rockey PH, Fantel JD: Discriminatory aspects of preemployment screening. Low back x-ray examinations in the railroad industry. American J of Law and Medicine 5(3):197-214.
31. American Occupational Medical Association: Guidelines for use of routine x-ray examinations in occupational medicine. J of Occup Med 21:500-502, 1979.

32. Houston CS: Pre-employment radiographs of lumbar spine. (Editorial). J Canad Assoc Radiol 28:170, 1977.
33. Macdonald EB, Porter R, Hibbert C, Hart J: The relationship between spinal canal diameter and back pain in coal miners. J of Occup Med 26(1):23-27, 1984.
34. NIOSH: A work practice guide for manual lifting. Technical Report #81-122, U.S. Department of Health and Human Services. NIOSH. Cincinnati, Ohio, 1981.
35. Chaffin DB: Human strength capability and low back pain. J Occup Med 16(4):248-253, 1974.
36. Chaffin DB, Herrin GD, Keyserling WM: Pre-employment strength testing. An updated position. J of Occup Med 20(6):403-408, 1978.
37. Keyserling WM, Herrin GD, Chaffin DB: Isometric strength testing as a means of controlling medical incidents on strenuous jobs. J of Occup Med 22(5):332-336, 1980.
38. Keyserling WM, Herrin GD, Chaffin DB, et al: Establishing an industrial strength testing program. Am Ind Hyg Assoc J, October 1980. pp 730-736.
39. Chaffin DB, Andersson G: Occupational Biomechanics. John Wiley & Sons, New York, 1984.
40. Troup JDG, Foreman TK, Baxter CE, Brown D: The perception of back pain and the role of psychophysical tests of lifting capacity. Spine 12(7):645-657, 1987.
41. Griffin AB, Troup JDG, Lloyed DCEF: Tests of lifting and handling capacity: Their reapeatability and relationship to back symptoms. Ergonomics 27:305-320, 1984.
42. Hanman B: Physical capacities and job placement. Nordisk Rotogravyr, Stockholm, 1951.
43. Fleishman EA: Toward a taxonomy of human performance. American Psychology 30:1127-1149, 1975.
44. Snook SH: Approaches to preplacement testing and selection of workers. Ergonomics 30(2):241-247, 1987.
45. Scholz H, Sieber W: Arbeibgestaltung und muskelermudung, ROM rhmerlwand hettinger Th RKW. Arbeitsphysiologie-Arbeitspsychologie, Berlin, Beith Vertried, 1963.
46. Andersson BJG, Ortengren R, Nachemson AL, Elfstrom G, Broman H: The sitting posture: an electromyographic and discometric study. Orthop Clinics of North America 6:105-120, 1975.
47. Mital A, Fard HF: Psychophysical and physiological responses to lifting symmetrical and asymmetrical loads symmetrically and asymmetrically. Ergonomics 29(10)1263-1272, 1986.
48. Chaffin DB, etal.: Workplace Design. In Pope MII, Frymoyer JW, (Eds.): Occupational Low Back Pain,Praegee, 1984.

49. Troup JDG: Driver's back pain and its prevention. A review of the postural, vibratory and muscular factors, together with the problem of transmitted road-shock. Applied Ergonomics, Dec:207-214, 1978.
50. Bentson JD: Control of low back pain in industry through ergonomic redesign of manual materials handling tasks. In Karwowski W (eds): Trends in Ergonomics/Human Factors III. Amsterdam, North Holland, 1986.
51. Westgaard RH, Aaras A: The effect of improved workplace design on the develpment of work-related musculoskeletal illnesses. Appl Ergonomics 16:91, 1985.
52. Dul J, Hildebrandt VH: Ergonomic guidelines for the prevention of low back pain at the workplace. Ergonomics 30(2):419-429, 1987.
53. Anderson CK, Chaffin DB: A biomechanical evaluation of five lifting techniques. Applied Ergonomics 17:2, 1986.
54. Garg A, Herrin GD: Stoop or squat: a biomechanical and metabolic evaluation. AIIE Transactions 11:293, 1979.
55. Brown JR: Lifting as an industrial hazard. Labour Safety Council of Ontario, Ontario Dept of Labour, Toronto, 1971.
56. U.S. Department of Health and Human Services: Work practices guide for manual lifting. DHHS(NIOSH) Publication No. 81-122, March, 1981.
57. Glover JR: Prevention of back pain. In Jayson M (ed): The Lumbar Spine and Back Pain. New York, Grune and Stratton, 1976.
58. Miller RL: Bend your knees! Nat Safety News. May, 1977, p 57.
59. Dehlin O, Hedenrud B, Horal J: Back symptoms in nursing aides in a geriatric hospital. Scand J Rehab Med 8:47, 1976.
60. Locke JC: Stretching away from back pain, injury. Occup Health & Safety, July:8-13, 1983.
61. Cady LD, Bischoff DP, O'Connell ER, et al: Strength and fitness and subsequent back injuries in firefighters. J Occup Med 21:269, 1979.
62. Cady LD, Thomas PC, Karwasky RJ: Program for increasing health and physical fitness of firefighters. J Occup Med 27:110, 1985.
63. Nutter P: Aerobic exercise in the treatment and prevention of low back pain. Occup Med: State of the Art Reviews 3(1):137-155, 1988.
64. Morris A: Program compliance key to preventing low back injuries. Occup Health & Safety, March:44-47, 1984.
65. Tomer GM, Oson CN: Back injury prevention training makes dollars and sense. Nat Safety News. Jan:36-39, 1984.
66. Fitzler SL, Berger RA: Chelsea back program: One year later. Occup Health & Safety 52(7):52-54, 1983.
67. Health Insurance Association of America: Your guide to wellness at the worksite. Washington D.C., 1983, p 10.

68. Pilcher OJ: Personal correspondence to Snook SH. February 9, 1979. From Snook SH: Approaches to the control of back pain in industry: Job design, job placement and education/training. Occup Med: State of the Art Reviews 3(1):45-59, 1988.
69. Johnson CD: Safety forum. Ind Safety Prod News. June 21, 1981.
70. Snook SH: Approaches to the control of back pain in industry: Job design, job placement and education/training. Occup Med: State of the Art Reviews 3(1):45-56, 1988.
71. McGill CM: Industrial back problems: a control program. J Occup Med 10:174, 1968.
72. Rosen NB: Treating the many facets of pain. Business & Health. May 7, 1986.

CHAPTER 6

The Consequences of Chronic Low Back Pain

Introduction

When an acute back injury is left unresolved by treatment and the natural healing process, the pain that was once restricted to the lumbar spine often initiates a psychological transformation in the individual as he or she confronts the fear and frustration of prolonged pain with no relief in sight. What was once an acute problem gradually becomes intractable pain, as the patient tries to maintain his composure amidst conflicting feelings of dependence, resentment, depression, and increasingly neurotic personality traits. Sleep disturbance, appetite changes, decreased libido, impaired concentration and irritability are some of the milder behavioral changes commonly associated with a chronic back condition. Whereas acute pain lasts no more than 3 to 6 months depending on the doctor's classification preference, a chronic condition refers to constant pain lasting a minimum of six months duration. Aronoff distinguishes between acute and chronic pain in the following manner: Acute pain is biologically useful and often reflects an underlying disorder which can usually be relieved by narcotic, physical or surgical treatments. In chronic pain syndromes, pain no longer serves an adaptive purpose and often becomes the disease. Thus, chronic pain, chronic disability, and chronic illness behavior become increasingly disassociated from their original physical basis, and resistant to traditional medical treatment [1].

While the link between psychological disturbance and chronic low back pain is generally accepted, whether such disturbances are the cause or result of the chronicity is not yet clear. On one side of the debate are the proponents of the "psychosomatic" model. The theory suggests that certain emotional reactions associated with pain can and frequently do cause alterations of body functions that can either aggravate existing pain or cause new pain to develop. The classic case of psychosomatic back pain is muscle spasm (see Etiology chapter). What began as a mild back spasm spirals into a vicious pain-tension cycle wherein anxiety causes further tension of the muscles, increasing anxiety still more, which in turn produces more muscular tension, stress and ever-increasing levels of pain. With time, more and more situations may elicit pain and anxiety, the end result being the chronic stimulation of the nervous system, greater dependence on medication, muscular atrophy and increasing disability. Ultimately, this sequence of circumstances can perpetuate pain long after the original noxious stimulus has healed. Others believe that neurosis is the product of protracted back disability.

In an effort to further an understanding of the roles that psychologic and physiologic factors play in the manifestation of pain, the medical profession has developed two general classifications that distinguish the causes of reported pain. If the probable cause of pain is identified by imaging technology or exhibits characteristics that falls into known or readily classifiable patterns, the cause of pain is considered "organic." Those cases which lack observable physical evidence of pathology after imaging or neurological examination are dubbed "non-organic," "psychogenic" or "functional." It is quite rare that a back case is purely physiologic or psychologic – the two realms are nearly always integrated together in the perception of and reaction to pain.

Regardless of whether neurosis is primary or secondary to chronicity, pain has both physical and emotional components that affect one's perception and reaction to injury or illness. Unless both aspects of back pain are confronted, accurate diagnosis and suitable treatment of the chronic patient is virtually impossible. All too often, the background and training of physicians encourages a very strong emphasis on the anatomical, physiological and neurological aspects of the pain complaint, while neglecting the patient's emotional status. Medicine teaches a theory of pain wherein the extent of tissue damage determines the intensity of the pain, and therefore the experience of pain. However, the research to be described below clearly indicates that pain is not simply a function of organic pathology.

Psychological Abnormalities

Concerning the focus on physical etiology which can almost be described as 'tunnel vision', Waddell remarks: "Medical treatment may in theory be prescribed for physical indications, but in practice both conservative and surgical treatment for a poorly understood condition such as low-back pain is determined to a much greater extent than most physicians realize or would like to admit by the patient's distress and illness behavior (i.e. psychological abnormality). . . . Medical decisions about conservative and surgical treatment are influenced more by distress and illness behavior than by physical indications" [2]. Instead of the traditional emphasis on noxious stimuli, the most effective management approach will not ignore the environmental context of chronic pain, especially critical to those circumstances when an organic complaint may be only a symptom of a greater social and psychological disturbance.

As the reader will discover in the studies to follow, many chronic back pain sufferers magnify the painful effects of their pathology to such a disproportionate degree that pain attributed to the underlying physical problem is overwhelmed by psychological distress. In Finneson's experience, the psychoneurotic person is often prone to seize upon an ache or pain and so distort and exaggerate it that the major symptom complex he eventually manifests can hardly be recognized in relationship to the original pain [3]. The failure of the clinician to account for the presence of psychological disturbance and evaluate the extent to which a neurotic condition influences the report of pain can lead to a misinterpretation of diagnostic data and improper treatment. The consequences of accepting a pain complaint at face value, warns Sternbach, can lead to less than favorable results for both doctor and patient: "The patient who overstates the intensity of pain may be over-treated, whereas those who understate it may suffer needlessly" [4]. These problems encouraged the development of a multidisciplenary approach to the diagnosis and management of chronic back pain which emphasized an awareness of the complex interaction between physiologic- and psychologic-induced pain.

An important tool utilized by the medical profession to help clarify the psychological nature of pain and aid in the selection of patients emotionally suited to various treatment modalities (especially surgery) is the personality test. The most commonly used tests include the Minnesota Multiphasic Personality Inventory (MMPI), the Eysenck Personality Inventory, the Beck Depression Inventory, the Zung Depression Scale and the McGill Pain Questionaire. Such tests deal primarily with interpersonal, social, and vocational areas, providing the doctor with a social context in which to evaluate the patient's problem. In the absence of diagnosable organic disease, this sort of information can be instrumental in measuring the influence of psychiatric factors involved with the alleged back illness.

The remainder of this section will discuss the psychology of chronic low back pain in terms of the personality traits most frequently associated with the condition, as indicated by various psychological tests and other data, both theoretical and empirical. In addition, attention will be paid to the predictive powers of the tests in assessing treatment outcome. During the course of evaluating the material, the reader may be tempted to dismiss the data as too theoretical, too far removed from medical research, and irrelevant to the study of industrial low back pain. Perhaps for the layman, but the surgeon may not wish to undertake a potentially irreversible operation without knowing something about the psychological state of the patient. Such information may assist the surgeon in deciding which patients are more likely to respond favorably to medical therapy or psychotherapeutic intervention.

Since the MMPI is by far the most commonly used personality assessment tool, the reader should be introduced to the structure, mechanics and scoring methods of the test to knowledgably evaluate the data. Composed of 556 true-false items and a list of 41 critical items (some of which may indicate serious behavioral disturbance), the test takes one to two hours. The basic test profile consists of three validity scales and ten clinical scales. Each scale has an average value of 50 and a standard deviation of 10. Scores above 70 occur in less than 2.5% of the normal population. Hypochondriasis, depression, and hysteria are the traits most commonly associated with chronic back pain and generally considered the most informative portion of the test, although current statistical analysis has increased the significance of the other clinical scales. The remaining personality indeces are psychopathic deviation, masculinity/femininity, paranoia, psychasthenia, schizophrenia, hypomania, and social introversion. The hypochondria scale is based upon multiple somatic complaints in the absence of organic etiology, related almost entirely to preoccupation with physical health. The depression scale measures the intensity of depressed moods, while hysteria measures the degree of pain complaint lacking an organic basis.

Once the MMPI has been completed, the "neurotic triad" (Hypochondriasis, Depression, and Hysteria scales) can be charted and compared to various configurations indicative of various states of psychological disturbance. According to Peterson, the most constructive use of the MMPI is as an indicator of the likelihood of certain thoughts, feelings, and behaviors that have particular relevance to pain [5]. This indicator would consider the likelihood of a patient experiencing bodily distress and complaining about a given incident. The 'Conversion V' is probably the best known configuration, patterned after a moderately high depression level sandwiched in between abnormally high hypochondria and hysteria levels. Research has indicated that psychological problems are observed in patients showing the classical conversion pattern. Not surprisingly, this configuration is considered predictive of a poor response to any medical treatment, most notably surgical intervention [6].

While few researchers would dispute the significance of the 'neurotic triad' as a generalized psychological portrait, there is little consensus over specific interpretation and application of the MMPI patterns. The test does have some notable drawbacks which must be considered by the physician. Watkins comments: "The MMPI is the state of the patient only at the time of the examination. It is doubtful that our common malady of backache becomes chronic only according to personality types. It may only mean that if the pain is of a certain intensity of character, and the loss of function of a certain duration or type, then the personality will be affected"[7]. This is significant because detailed information about each patient's personality complex can aid the the doctor in deciding which treatment modalities are most appropriate to a given psychopathological situation. For example, most would argue that a patient having undergone multiple laminectomies and demonstrating a 'Conversion V' profile on the MMPI is a very poor candidate for spinal fusion. The surgeon might find that manipulating certain behavioral elements that interact between the patient and his environment would help reduce the tremendous distress the patient feels. If this were the case, efforts could be made to address the psychological component of pain through treatments such as relaxation training techniques, EMG biofeedback, anti-depressant medication or other psychotherapeutic techniques that encourage a positive reinforcement to get better. While these modalities will be discussed at length in the next section, one cannot talk of treatment without first describing the actual psychologic abnormalities.

The association of depression and chronic pain has been examined by a number of authors but the exact relationship is unclear. A close linkage between the state of depression and the experience of bodily pain is described throughout the literature. The depressive symptoms of the chronic pain patient tend to be viewed as the consequence of physical suffering from which there appears to be no relief. Yet some speculate that depression can be traced beyond the organic lesion (if it exists at all) to the social environment of the patient. Indeed, Pilowsky et al. have described the typical chronic pain patient in terms of the following characteristics: 1. a hypochondriacal preoccupation; 2. rejection of any suggestion that their pain is a result of a psychological factors; 3. admission that they have difficulty in expressing their feelings to other people; 4. description of themselves as frequently sad or anxious as a result of their pain; and 5. strong reluctance to acknowledge any life problems [8].

Additionally, Engle believes individuals most prone to chronic pain tend to show the following traits: a prominence of guilt, a history of suffering, defeat, an intolerance of success, a strong aggressive drive that is not fulfilled, and the development of pain upon a loss or threatened loss [9]. The common denominator of both lists is the inability to recognize and verbalize one's feelings. Pain may become an acceptable way of saying "Now it's my turn to be taken care of!" The cumulative effect of these personality difficulties offers an interesting explanation of the MMPI 'Conversion V' configuration because it indicates how relatively low levels of depression can co-exist with constant back pain. Known as "masked depression," this paradoxical phenomenon occurs in many cases because suffering is experienced more through somatic pain rather than mental anguish. According to the theory, chronic pain is the somatic expression of an unresolved psychic pain caused by any combination of factors described above. As an example, consider Clawson's example of the housewife who, unable to control her husband or dominate the children in health, finds that through disability she is able to obtain companionship, love and attention that she sought unsuccessfully as a healthy wife and mother [10].

The reader should note that the preceding hypothesis dealing with the pain-prone personality explained through a psychoanalytic approach has not yet been subjected to an adequate test. Most of the research in this field is retrospective, usually uncontrolled, and is further characterized by serious methodological problems. While empirical evidence is sparse and not well elaborated, the greatest amount of evidence to support the theory is the relative pervasiveness of depression noted among populations of chronic pain patients. At the very least, these theories offer interesting suggestions about the development of chronic pain states and take into consideration psychological factors that purely somatic models tend to neglect.

The typical chronic back personality scenario compiled by Pilowsky [8] and Enge [19] describes what Waddel [12] terms "illness behavior." According to Waddell, the most important psychologic disturbance in low back pain is emotional distress. Distress is observed as disturbance of emotion and mood in which psychologic and physical symptoms occur, the equivalent of the "neurotic triad" (increased bodily awareness and depression) on the MMPI. Based upon his experience with 200 patients who underwent full clinical, physical and psychologic assessment, the author proposes that "illness behavior" is a considerably more accurate depiction of the chronic pain of the patient's emotional status than is it an approach in using personality tests like the MMPI. Rather than label the patients as neurotic, hypochondriac, hysterical or paranoid, the concept of illness behavior considers such traits as the cumulative outward manifestation of an underlying organic disease. While the concept could be considered as a simple change of language, illness behavior is neither judgemental, stigmatizing or misleading, unlike psychiatric terminology such as "hypochondria" or "hysteria." In other words, illness behavior is an expression of the individual's own perception of disturbed health, and as such it is neither legitimate or illegitimate. Overreaction to examination and superficial tenderness (two of eight inappropriate responses to physical examination) were noted as a "magnified presentation or communication of the severity of the patient's whole problem and of the need to do something about it" [2].

Magnification of mood-related attributes of pain among individuals with chronic back pain is consistent with a report by Leavitt et al. [11]. Investigating the association between descriptions of pain and psychological disturbance, back patients were assigned to three study groups on the basis of MMPI results. Those patients in Group 1 demonstrated the least psychopathology, with pain scores strikingly similar to pain scores produced by patients whose low back pain was associated with organic disease but who had no evidence of psychologic disturbance. Those in Group 3 showed the greatest number of MMPI elevations and presumably the most psychologic disturbance. Group 3 patients described their pain with the most intensity, involving a greater range of sensory and affective qualities. These patients admitted to a wide variety of symptoms, problems and feelings clearly psychiatric in origin. The significance of this data is explained in the author's concluding remarks: "An important implication of this pattern is that the pain complaint, itself, may well have detrimental effects on patient care and should not be used alone as a measure of treatment need... Thus the value of treatment may well depend as much upon affecting the psychological status of the patient as on providing appropriate forms of medical treatment."

Does the duration of chronic pain affect the psychological stability of the sufferer, or is the emotional experience of acute and chronic pain similar? Garron et al. examined the psychological aspects of chronic low back pain compared to the duration of pain, which ranged from recent onset to more than two years standing [12]. The 148 participants were organized into three groups according to pain duration: recent onset (0 to 6 months), relatively longstanding (6 to 24 months), and chronic (more than 24 months). Four personality questionnaires were used in the study. The MMPI was used to sample psychological and personality characteristics. The State Trait Anxiety Inventory (STAI) was used to differentiate between state and trait anxiety. The Multiple Affect Adjective Check List (MAACL) was used to differentiate among current states of anxiety, depression, and hostility. The Low Back Pain Questionnaire (LBPQ) was used to indicate whether the experience of the pain itself was affected by chronicity.

The results indicated that chronic low back pain leads to the development of psychological abnormality. Data from the MMPI showed a tendency to rise with increasing duration of pain. Those patients with pathology of recent onset were judged psychologically normal, while those with more chronic disability scored significantly higher on six of the MMPI scales, with peak scores on both the hysteria and hypochondria indexes. The authors interpreted this finding to mean that "the apparent psychopathology seen in patients with low back pain of long duration cannot be attributed solely to pre-existing personality characteristics." Interestingly, the mood scales of the STAI and MAACL did not increase with increasing chronicity, prompting speculation that "chronic pain may involve a psychopathologically heightened awareness of somatic functioning and perhaps other psychopathological changes in attitude, but not in subjective mood." The final noteworthy phenomenon was the absence of any changes in the perception of pain itself, as confirmed by the LBPQ scales. Thus, back pain in the chronic state is qualitatively similar to back pain in the acute state, suggesting that "the level of perceived disability associated with the back has not changed with time."

Other studies have investigated different aspects of the depression-chronic pain linkage. Sternbach et al. evaluated 68 patients with low back pain and observed significant elevation on the MMPI depression scale, prompting the author to conclude that the group was "clearly depressed, and their illness may be simply termed a psychophysiogical muscular-skeletal reaction with depression" [13]. A study of 16 moderately to severely depressed patients found 100% of them to have chronic pain complaints [14]. Treated with anti-depressant medication, a highly significant association was found between improvement of depression and reduction of pain. A similar observation was noted by Sternbach in a later study, noting a decrease in some indicators of psychopathology among patients whose pain had been relieved, implying that the psychopathology is the by-product of pain [15].

Yet some studies have indicated only a mild correlation between depression and chronic back pain, indicating that there is no agreement on how widely prevalent depression is among chronic pain sufferers. Merskey, for example, compared 100 psychiatric patients with pain to 65 pain-free controls and found that persistent pain had more pronounced correlation with hysteria and anxiety than with depression [16]. A report by Beals et al. noted "with passage of time following injury, patients increasingly elaborate and exaggerate their symptoms but are less truly depressed by their predicament,[17] " an analysis which could explain the 'Conversion V' configuration of mild depression and abnormal hysteria and hypochondria.

The Psychology of Organic (Structural) versus Functional Pain

Unlike the previous study by Waddell, one investigator is so convinced of a depressive component involved in chronic conditions that he has stated emphatically: "Whenever a patient complains of pain for which no organic basis can be found, the physician should suspect the presence of an underlying depression" [18]. On the surface, this bold statement seems like an excessive generalization. However, the reader will recall the Vallfors report from Sweden(discussed in the Epidemiology chapter) which noted a non-organic diagnosis in 70% of all chronic back patients examined [19]. Furthermore, these patients reported the greatest amount of dissatisfaction with their social and professional lives, and had a greater frequency of smoking, peptic ulcer, alcoholism, and disatisfaction with their co-workers. A more significant problem than establishing a strong association between depression and non-organic findings is the confirmation of depressive symptoms (often hidden) using personality tests. If such testing were to identify depressive symptoms with minimal error, the physician would then be able to terminate or continue physical treatment as soon as test results were available. Of course, the decision to discontinue medical treatment and begin psychotherapy hinges on accurate personality assessment.

However, whether or not the MMPI or other personality test can accurately distinguish between patients with and without organic evidence of pathology is a matter of great importance and a topic of intense controversy. Hanvik [20] reported that patients with functional pain were clearly more depressed and anxious than organic patients, based upon significantly elevated MMPI conversion scales (hypochondria, hysteria and depression) [20]. Additionally, the non-organic patients scored significantly higher on scales indicating impulsivity, anxiety and confusion. Freeman reported nearly identical results – functional patients showed higher profiles than organic patients on all scales, except for the impulsivity index [21]. The same trend was noted by Merskey et al, who reported that patients lacking organic lesions had considerably more evidence of unhappy childhood, premorbid personality problems and marital difficulties compared to patients with lesions of organic origin [22]. Other authors have noted similar patterns in MMPI data, yet they acknowledge that despite significant differences between functional and organic patients, there is so much overlap between the groups that the differences are not clinically useful. [23,24]

On the other side of the debate is that body of research which has not observed any appreciable differences in psychological distress among organic and functional patients. McCreary compared the MMPI scores of 42 organic back patients to 37 functional back patients and found that the functional group scored significantly higher on the "neurotic triad" scales, as well as three other scales [25]. However, the statistical level of significance for the differences was not as high as in the Hanvik or Freeman studies. While McCreary found higher depression and anxiety scores in the functional patients, the differences were calculated as not significant. In fact, the groups did not differ in terms of their reported overall intensity of pain or reported degree of functional limitation due to pain. Additionally, a significant degree of overlap between the group scores on the hysteria and hypochondria scales was noted. On each of these scales, approximately 25% to 30% of the functional patients scored below the average of the organic group and a similar percentage of organic patients scored above the average of the functional group.

Obviously, such a report does not support the view that patients lacking physical signs of pathology be labeled as "psychogenic" cases. Consistent with this finding, Woodforde used the Eysenck Personality Inventory to demonstrate that patients with pain of a physical origin were actually more anxious, depressed and subject to signs of neuroticism (more likely to experience emotional breakdown under stress) than a group of patients with non-organic pain [26]. Sternbach et al. analyzed the MMPI profiles of 81 patients with organic findings and 36 with no findings, and observed that the profiles were essentially the same. He concluded: "The clear psychophysiological profile displayed by both groups is apparently independent of whether or not physical findings are detected on examination" [27]. Several other investigations confirm this viewpoint, but will not be discussed here. Instead, the reader will be able to refer to this literature in the section dealing with compensation of back disability and the role that secondary gain plays in the psychology of organic and non-organic back pain.

Is a distinction between patients with functional and organic pain all that useful, in light of the literature's inability to demonstrate any differences in MMPI profiles? McCreary remarks: "Study of this distinction may help illuminate some basic theoretical issues concerning the nature of chronic pain, especially the relationship between the learning history and coping styles of pain patients and their physiologic processes... In addition, a study of this distinction may produce certain clinically useful guidelines for the matching of patients to maximally beneficial treatment" [25]. Hence, if a physician is able to identify the psychosomatic patient seeking a physical cure for psychological and interpersonal difficulties, such a distinction could be invaluable in the selection of possible treatment modalities. Since the distinction between functional and organic pain is directly related to the diagnosis of chronic pain, more information will be discussed on this topic in the following section dealing with the diagnosis and treatment of chronic low back pain.

Even if all the indications of functional illness are clearly manifest to the doctor, many are hesitant to label the patient with such a diagnosis. Finneson attributes this reluctance to several factors [3]. In many instances, neither the patient nor family will accept a diagnosis of non-organic disease, frequently dropping all relations with the doctor and seeking medical opinion and aid elsewhere. Secondly, a non-organic diagnosis might jeopardize the underwriting of full medical coverage by insurance companies. For example, insurance plans may attempt to avoid payment of the hospital and doctor bills. A third reason for the reticence of physicians to officially acknowledge a diagnosis of functional low back pain is observed in cases of pending litigation. "In medicolegal problems, mention of nonorganic symptoms is anathema to the patient's attorney, since this will weaken his bargaining position at settlement or in court." Such a diagnosis could jeopardize the physician's future involvement in the treatment of the patient, not to mention any involvement in deposition or expert testimony on behalf of the plaintiff. Finally, most doctors are also concerned about erroneously considering the patient's complaint as non-organic in the presence of organic disease.

Diagnosis Of Psychogenic Pain

The diagnosis of non-specific low back pain, completely lacking in physical evidence of pathology, defies conventional medical analysis. Low back pain often escapes detection by the most sensitive imaging technology and physical examinations. Finneson states: "The evaluation of pain for treatment is made difficult by the fact that pain is an almost entirely subjective phenomenon. It is especially difficult to differentiate organic from psychic factors. The problem is further complicated because in most, if not all patients, both factors contribute to the final expression of pain. Furthermore, the proportion of contribution by the somatic and psychic spheres changes constantly. It is in this area of diagnosis that the art of the physician is most severely challenged and is almost impossible to subject to quantitative evaluation and criticism" [3].

A careful history and physical examination are the principal factors in establishing a diagnosis of physogenic pain syndrome and its severity. Once an organic etiology has been ruled out, there are several indicators that are helpful in determining the psychosocial aspects of chronic pain. In addition to the more obvious personality traits such as depression and hypochondria discussed above, the observant physician should recognize the significance of the following factors:

1. A dramatic description of pain that clearly does not fit the clinical experience. The use of such adjectives as "shooting, punishing, wretched, sickening, crushing, drilling " or a comment like "the pain was like a knife stabbed into my back" could be a reflection of psychiatric disorder. Research has indicated that patients with psychological disturbance use more words in their description of pain and distribute these words over more pain factors, regardless of the organicity of their condition [11]. Additionally, symptoms described in terms that are vague, ill-localized and lack the normal relationships to time, physical activity, and anatomy are commonly associated with psychologic features [28]. A patient claiming to have experienced pain and/or numbness throughout his entire leg or pain at the tip of the tail-bone is an example of inappropriate symptoms.
2. Physical findings that are inconsistent with the complaint. According to Clawson, this is most commonly seen in the over-reaction to light touch or a jerking reaction to requests to flex or extend the spine or while conducting straight-leg-raising examinations [10]. Such a patient may also be able to tolerate tests when distracted that cannot be tolerated when the patient is concentrating on what the examiner is doing.
3. A past history of violence, pain, or chronic disease in the family is positively correlated with injury or disease of the individual.
4. An indication that many other organic systems are involved in addition to the low back problem. As symptoms from one system clear, symptoms from a new system will appear after a short period of time. The denial of the patient that problems other than the specific injury or illness could be contributing to the etiology of the lumbar pathology is a classic trait among psychologically disturbed patients. These signs are consistent with hypochondria, also characterized by a hostile attitude toward the many physicians they have visited in the past for other ailments lacking objective findings. In addition to back pain, the hypochondriac usually manifests symptoms of nervousness, irritability, insomnia, and shortness of breath, all of which may be aggravated by increased intensity of the backache.
5. Chronic anxiety, characterized by an irritable, anxious, overreactive and tense nature. These traits are commonly accompanied by painful back spasms, caused by the pain-tension cycle discussed earlier in the section.
6. Dependency on medication, drugs or alcohol.

7. Financial compensation, pending litigation or other secondary gain factors may be related to non-organic pathology and psychological disorders. Clawson notes that the patient's ability to manipulate the environment to suit his emotional and physical needs provide a powerful incentive to remain in a chronically injured state. Thus, secondary gain need not be financial, but can range from obtaining the love and attention of family or friends to gaining an "honorable and socially acceptable retreat from a vexatious task, without scorn or criticism from either fellow workers or family." The secondary gain issue will be discussed in much greater detail in the succeeding section.

8. Cultural factors can also play a part in psychogenic pain. For example, studies have revealed differences of response to illness and pain among very ethnic groups. Patients of Italian or Jewish origin were found to express pain more vividly and have a lower pain threshold, compared to Irish, English and German Americans who were considered less demonstrative.

9. Family influence is another environmental factor. Calliet notes: "The relationship of family members with regard to their support or their condemnation may contribute to the severity of the patient's complaints about the alleged incapacity" [29]. The operative mechanism reinforcing illness behavior in this case is the family members who derive satisfaction from the role of caretaker, and the patient who receives love and attention in return for his continued disability. Divorce, a death in the family, the loss of a job, or other crises are all relevant social factors which can contribute to a chronic back ailment.

Psychological Treatment

The failure of an acute back injury or illness to respond to conventional therapy after several months amidst continuing indications of non-organic symptoms requires a change in treatment focus -- from physical to psychological. Assuming that the patient remains unresponsive to traditional pain management techniques, an approach that emphasizes the behavioral elements of pain is warranted, and endorsed by the vast majority of current medical and psychological research. The physician that differentiates pain caused by tissue damage from pain caused by an underlying psychologic disability, psychosomatic factors, or maladaptive behavioral patterns is undoubtedly going to be more successful in treating the patient than is the doctor who treats only the cause of pain while neglecting the symptoms entirely. In order to maximize the efficacy of treatment it is vital that the physician consider back pain as a set of behaviors that include such variables as medication intake, activity levels, mood and pain ratings.

Psychological treatment can be classified into three fundamental categories: operant, relaxation (respondent), and cognitive. Each approach will be discussed in terms of explanatory models, treatment objectives, the logic of intervention, theoretical application and efficacy.

Operant Treatment

Operant conditioning procedures are designed to decrease the frequency of pain behavior and increase the frequency of healthy behavior through positive and negative social reinforcement. Linton defines the approach in this manner: "From the operant viewpoint, pain is a set of overt responses (eg medication taking, limping, pain reports) which can be controlled by reinforcers (eg attention, medications, etc) if the reinforcers are given contingent on the pain behaviors" [30]. The objectives are three-fold: the extinction of pain behaviors such as moaning or asking for sympathy by the withdrawal of attention and/or medication; the promotion of wellness behavior; and the maintenance of these changes in the patient's natural environment through the active involvement of family and friends.

Fordyce is credited with the development of operant treatment, and most operant programs are modeled after his theory of chronic pain [31]. These programs concentrate on decreasing medication intake, pain levels and pain behavior, and increasing more constructive behavior. For example, because medication is seen as a reward for continued pain (acting as a positive reinforcer), medication is switched from a pain-contingent ("as-needed") to time-contingent basis, conforming to a specific time schedule. A reduction in drug dependency is achieved by serving the patient progressively smaller doses in a "pain cocktail." The "cocktail" becomes increasingly diluted by the vehicle, until the patient withdraws from the medicine all together. Physical rehabilitation is attained through the reinforcement of activity levels with lavish social praise and rest, while family and friends are encouraged by the physician to be socially unresponsive to complaints of pain or discomfort. The limitations of the operant approach include high expense and prolonged work absence.

As for the efficacy of these procedures, Fordyce examined the comparative effects of traditional versus operant methods in the early management of acute back injury [31]. Patients with back pain of less than two days were randomly assigned to one of the two treatment groups. The traditional therapy group received treatment on a pain-contingent basis. Prescribed analgesics were taken on an as-needed basis, while exercise and activity limits were undertaken according to the principle of "let pain be your guide." This treatment philosophy differed markedly from the operant therapy group, which was administered analgesics at fixed time intervals. Activity limits ended when a specified time interval had elapsed, while exercises were performed with a preset number of repetitions.

Results were tabulated according to post-treatment vocational status (absenteeism due to pain), health care utilization (including reliance on medication, doctor visits, and hospitalization), self-reported disability, self-reported pain, and activity ability. At a six-week follow-up, there were no significant differences between the two modalities in vocational status or in dependence on pain medication. However, at 9 to 12 months post-treatment, differences were clearly apparent. Patients treated according to conventional therapy principles were significantly more impaired than those patients treated with operant methods, as evidenced by all of the data indices except vocational status. Fordyce remarks: "The central point of these findings seems to be that the prevention of chronicity in recent-onset back pain is furthered by distinguishing between pain and healing and designing regimens based on healing, not report of pain."

Consistent with the experience of Fordyce, a review of 15 studies by Linton demonstrated increases in activity levels, moderate decreases of subjective pain ratings and significant medication reduction in nearly all reports [30]. However, none of the studies were able to reduce pain below a rating of 4 on a 0 to 10 scale, meaning that patients still experienced considerable pain. It should be emphasized that only three studies in this group had control conditions of any type, thus it is impossible to attribute progress to the specific treatment. Also, rejection, refusal, and drop-out rates were often high, some studies evaluating as few as 40% of patients considered for treatment. Finally, no data comparing the operant approach with other treatment programs was reported.

Anderson et al. [32] found that nearly three-quarters of their study group reported leading normal lives at follow up ranging from six months to seven years. Unfortunately, the study is utterly inconclusive because no definition is offered to describe "normal" and only 34 of 130 patients were actually treated, while only 24 of this group were followed up. Cairns et al. confirmed the finding in a different study, reporting that 74% of the patients had stopped reliance on the health care system for their back problem [33]. Despite the methodological problems of most of these studies, Turk et al. [34] believe there is reason to be optimistic about the operant approach: "Given the fact that these patients usually had long-standing pain problems, often underwent multiple surgeries and had not profited from medical interventions, the results look quite promising albeit preliminary" [34].

The Relaxation Approach — EMG Biofeedback

Electromyographic activity within the back muscles has been discussed at length in both the epidemiology and diagnosis chapters. In those sections, it was noted that abnormally high levels of EMG activity during positions of rest and exertion may be a means of identifying sites of tissue inflammation and pathological disorder. Increased EMG activity can be attributed to the abnormal postures assumed in response to pain, with the trunk bent forward, shoulders rounded, and pelvis rotated. Some have also linked increased EMG levels to the initiation of aggressive impulses or anxiety-provoking conflicts, and decreased EMG activity to verbalization of fantasies, especially fantasies regarding flight from conflicts [35]. For instance, Holmes et al. reported that neurotic patients with back pain demonstrated generalized muscular hyperactivity during movement or during interviews that provoked the expression of conflicts and feeling of hostility [36]. The same observation was noted by Dorpat et al. [37], who found increased EMG activity during interviews that addressed personal conflicts, particularly feelings of hostility, guilt and frustration [37]. The reader will remember that these are precisely the same feelings discussed in the psychology section, which act as a catalyst in transforming psychic pain to physical pain.

Assuming that elevated levels of paraspinal contraction contribute to back pain, a treatment modality was developed that utilized EMG biofeedback to interrupt the viscious circle of pain-tension-pain and replace muscular overreaction with relaxation. Treatment emphasizes the role that the patient can play in reducing muscle tension and psychological stress as a means of controlling the pain. The typical treatment program provides the patient with a model of the relationship between tension and pain, after which EMG biofeedback is provided either from the scalp muscles or from the back muscles. The number of sessions commonly ranges from 1 to 20 with the biofeedback lasting from 2.5 minutes to 45 minutes.

Unfortunately, there is no concrete scientific evidence to support the assumed EMG reduction-pain reduction linkage. According to Turk et al. at least nine studies have reported significant reductions in pain intensity and/or frequency at post-treatment, while in at least five other studies the pain was not altered [34]. Most investigations have included supplementary treatment in addition to biofeedback, typically relaxation training, physical therapy and medication. This is not to suggest that EMG biofeedback can not be effective, for as many of the preceding reports have indicated, the placebo effects of such treatments can be substantial. After a review of the recent literature pertaining to biofeedback, Turk et al. concluded: "Although there are considerable methodological and design problems involved in the majority of the EMG biofeedback studies with chronic back pain, the fact that only controlled studies report similar, favorable results, makes EMG biofeedback appear a promising treatment modality for chronic back pain. EMG biofeedback combined with relaxation training or relaxation training alone may also be useful treatment modalities that deserve further consideration."

Nouwen conducted one of the few controlled trials investigating the efficacy of standing EMG biofeedback among 20 low back patients randomly assigned to treatment or non-treatment groups [38]. All subjects presented a pain history greater than six months, with no indications that pain was caused by spinal or other organic disturbances. Results were based on a daily log completed by the patient for a period of nine weeks — three weeks before, three weeks during, and three weeks after treatment. Pain intensity was recorded on a five-point scale each waking hour of the day. Each of the 15 treatment sessions were divided into three stages: EMG recording without biofeedback (pretreatment trials), biofeedback treatment (during which the patients were told to reduce EMG activity without changing posture), and EMG recording without feedback (post-treatment trials).

Nouwen found that the low back patients with relatively high standing paraspinal EMG were able to reduce these levels using biofeedback training. Despite the EMG reductions, no decrease in pain was reported, indicating that the reduction of paraspinal EMG during a painful posture is not necessarily related to pain decreases. At the time of the article's publication (1983), only one other controlled experiment (also by Nouwen) using similar biofeedback procedures, confirmed that standing paraspinal EMG reduction via biofeedback was unrelated to pain outcome [39]. In this earlier study, EMG biofeedback was compared with electrotherapy and a placebo. While only low back patients who received EMG treatment showed significantly lower levels of standing paraspinal EMG, both EMG and electrotherapy groups demonstrated similar pain decreases, as compared to the no-treatment control group in which no significant changes were observed. Nouwen admits that his findings contrast markedly with the observations of Jones et al, who describe a case study where reduction of low back pain was also accompanied by increases in range of motion, all as a result of EMG biofeedback [40].

Unlike the preceding report, a simultaneous reduction in EMG and back pain was observed by Flor et al, under test conditions very similar to Nouwen's report [41]. In this trial, 24 patients were randomly assigned to groups receiving EMG biofeedback, a credible pseudotherapy, and conventional medical treatment during a four week inpatient stay. The EMG group was assigned to practice relaxation at home, with a list of recommended cues for relaxation including muscular and emotional tension, and periods of pain. All cases were chronic back conditions of more than six months duration, with little or no minor degenerative changes of the vertebrae. The biofeedback training was composed of 12 sessions, with 20 minute training and 7 minute pre- and post-treatment evaluation. Outcome measures were interpreted in terms of a daily pain index kept by the patient in a diary, in addition to a questionnaire of pain-related positive and negative cognitions.

The study indicated that EMG biofeedback was more effective than either placebo or medical treatment. The EMG levels showed a significant decline only in the biofeedback group, while reduction in EMG levels was positively correlated with the reduction in the pain index from pre- and post-treatment. The post-treatment questionnaire revealed that the biofeedback group was more pleased with therapy than the other two groups, the patients in the control group being the least content. Those treated with EMG biofeedback were also "more convinced that they could control pain themselves, that they could relax better, that they could transfer their knowledge into their everyday lives, and they were also more optimistic about the duration of their therapeutic success." Interestingly enough, the examinations of the different dimensions of pain indicated that the benefits of biofeedback did not affect the sensory component of the pain experience, but instead worked primarily through the cognitive-evaluative and affective-motivational components of pain. This finding contradicts the fundamental logic that EMG treatment will lead to reduced muscle tension, and should involve the sensory mechanism. The report highlights the significant role that psychosocial stress (as discussed in the epidemiology chapter) plays in the preservation of chronic low back pain, illustrating the psychological benefit that biofeedback provides in the reduction of both EMG levels and pain.

The Cognitive-Behavioral Approach

The purpose of the cognitive approach is to ameliorate chronic pain at the level of perception, suffering and pain behavior[5]. This approach views pain as an experience mediated by cognitions. Because pain is a subjective experience, treatment at the cognitive level is considered useful in altering maladaptive thoughts, feelings, and behaviors, thereby changing the experience of pain. While the source of physical pain is not directly addressed, modifying cognitions with coping strategies such as hypnosis might reduce pain levels and provide the patient with a more effective method of pain management.

Reducing the patient's sense of helplessness and hopelessness is achieved by a variety of techniques. Education of the patient in the multidimensional aspects of pain is considered essential to enlisting the patient's active participation, and fundamental to the introduction of a more optimistic outlook. Additionally, most patients tend to have a very unsophisticated model of pain. Many are convinced that if the pain is not in their back than it must be in their head. Once an understanding of the physiologic and psychologic components of chronic pain is achieved, the patient is actively encouraged to adopt a new model of pain. Maintenance of this new attitude toward pain is aided by goal-setting. Patients are encouraged to achieve positive goals such as learning to be calm and relaxed, rather than eliminating problems such as mastering pain or eliminating it entirely. Instead, coping better, handling anxiety and depression, and adapting to necessary restrictions in occupation or activity are suggested as more realistic [42].

If these concepts and recommendations sound somewhat nebulous, the empirical evidence confirms that cognitive-behavioral modification is much better in theory than in practice. A review of five studies revealed "little evidence demonstrating that cognitive strategies are effective in the treatment of chronic pain or that they are the treatment of choice.... A lack of studies in combination with poor designs and the confounding of cognitive with noncognitive treatments prevents us from drawing any firm conclusions: clinical validity has not yet been really tested." For example, Cohen et al. compared cognitive-behavioral therapy to physical therapy in a sample of chronic back patients [43]. The ten-week cognitive program consisted of personal effectiveness training, education, relaxation, positive self-talk and activity increase. At the end of the treatment period, the physical therapy group showed a marginal increase in back control, no change in general activity, and little pain reduction. Patients in the cognitive-behavioral group reported subjectively more social and physical activity (unsubstantiated by diary data) and no change in pain.

On the other hand, Turner observed the opposite trend in a study which randomly assigned chronic low back pain patients to progressive-relaxation training, cognitive-behavioral therapy, or a waiting list group [44]. All 36 patients had suffered low back pain for at least six months. Cognition modification emphasized working toward individual goals, identifying the patient's cognitive and affective responses to pain, and learning to use relaxation and imagery techniques and coping self-statements to deal with pain and stress. At post-treatment, the condition of the waiting list patients was the same or had deteriorated with respect to self-rated pain severity, depression, and disability. Both relaxation-training and cognitive-behavioral therapy patients improved significantly on all indicators. At a one-month follow-up, the cognitive patients reported greater improvement than their counterparts in the ability to tolerate pain and participate in normal activities, while the relaxation-trained patients showed increased pain ratings, almost to the pre-treatment level. Long-term results from a follow-up 18 to 24 months post-treatment revealed that both patient groups had greatly decreased health care use and decreased pain intensity, with no significant differences between the two conditions.

Multimodal Treatment

Because pain is influenced by a large number of interacting variables, the multimodal approach seeks to maximize improvement by utilizing a combination of several treatment techniques. The three techniques discussed thusfar (operant, relaxation, and cognitive) are commonly integrated within the same treatment regimen, which might also include any number of other miscellaneous conservative modalities. A multimodal response to chronic back pain is in fact the rule rather than the exception, as only a handful of studies have evaluated the efficacy of treatment in a "vacuum" devoid of any other therapeutic techniques. Multimodal treatment of chronic pain is most commonly seen in pain clinics or centers. As Aronoff describes it, a pain clinic offers "multidisciplenary evaluation and treatment using an integrated pain team approach to modify pain and drug seeking behavior and to interrupt the disability process" [45]. Directly related to these goals are improvement of the patient's quality of life, reduction of suffering, assistance in returning to a functional and productive lifestyle, and reduced dependence on the health care system. In meeting these objectives, the multidisciplinary setting has the advantage of a team approach, usually including medicine, psychiatry, psychology, social services, nursing, physical therapy, and vocational counseling. Each discipline is best able to elicit and address the specific causes that add up to an individual's pain problem.

Most investigators report considerable improvement at discharge and follow-up. The typical report documents significant medication reduction, improved ability to cope with pain, improved physical functioning, and reduced pain. Perhaps the most favorable results were observed by Gottleib et al, who implemented an inpatient program emphasizing a cognitive perspective which also included stress management, biofeedback, psychological counseling, assertiveness training, self-regulated medication reduction, patient participation in case conferences, physical therapy, vocational rehabilitation and education. The report found 79% of the patients showing unrestricted physical functioning at discharge, and 95% with adequate vocational rehabilitation (working and training) at one month follow-up. At a six month follow-up, 46% of the group was contacted, 82% of which reported satisfactory vocational rehabilitation.

Interpretation of such results are difficult, considering that a "package" of treatments makes it impossible to determine the efficacy of any of the components or compare results among different studies. The paucity of controlled trials and the preliminary nature that characterizes much of the literature adds further confusion. Despite these methodological problems, the multimodal approach appears to be a legitimate alternative for treatment. Turk et al. comment: "Eclectic studies employing a number of interventions provide some evidence for the usefulness of comprehensive treatment programs. However, the lack of control groups, the lack of comprehensive pain assessment and the uncertainty about the effective components do not allow definite conclusions to be drawn. Here, too, a wide variety of patients have been treated with a lack of or widely divergent sample descriptions. It needs to determined which patients profit from what treatment" [34].

Compensation And Litigation

Thusfar, chronic back pain has been discussed in terms of the psychological variables commonly associated with the condition. The propensity for the chronic patient to experience pain in the absence of organic trauma is a primary reason explaining the frustrating inability of the physician to diagnose and treat the patient. While non-organic findings can be attributed to the complicated nature of lumbar anatomy or genuine psychologic disturbance, the role that compensation plays in the perpetuation of symptoms is without doubt vexing. Many within the medical community have argued that patients receiving disability payments or having litigation pending are less likely to benefit from any kind of intervention, especially in cases without organic evidence of injury. It is claimed that compensation (as well as other forms of secondary gain) provides a substantial incentive to complain of pain when it is not present, or exaggerate its severity in order to maximize damages or benefits. Thus, it is not surprising that the typical worker's compensation case has become the pariah among pain patients. In fact, this belief has led to the invention of the diagnostic entity known as "compensation neurosis," cynically defined as "a state of mind, born out of fear, kept alive by avarice, stimulated by lawyers, and cured by a verdict" [47]. These patients are commonly regarded as neurotics and malingerers. As Rothman indicates, "No stratagem could have been developed with a greater bias against a person's getting well than the system that so generously rewards a person for staying ill" [48].

Intuitively, it seems quite logical that the compensation status of a low-back injury may be strongly related to the presence or absence of organic disease signs and/or psychologic disturbance. One would consider this logic especially appropriate to the chronic back case, where a variety of behavioral, social, and economic factors have been shown to exist. For example, Snook [49] has found that patients receiving workers' compensation for back injuries were less likely to have objective findings or a definitive diagnosis than those with back injuries who were not receiving compensation [49].

Although some articles have documented evidence of poorer treatment outcome among patients receiving compensation, there is a growing body of evidence that patients who receive compensation are no different from patients who do not. The remainder of this section will examine why compensation is such a controversial topic among the medical, legal, and industrial communities. An emphasis will be placed on empirical evidence that supports or refutes the belief that the compensated patient is more likely than the non-compensated patient to: be more psychologically disturbed, suffer from a non-organic disease or injury, and fail to respond to a wide array of treatments.

The reader should exercise caution in formulating conclusions about the various studies to follow because most of them suffer from serious methodological problems. This is true not only for the body of research dedicated to chronic pain, but every aspect of back pain research discussed in this book — Epidemiology, Etiology, Treatment, Diagnosis, and Prevention. Among the various methodologic flaws encountered in the literature are the following [1]:

1. lack of comparison and control groups
2. use of subjective self-report measures of treatment outcome
3. use of outcome measures with questionable reliability and validity

4. dependence on mailed questionnaires
5. failure to use standardized testing instruments
6. lack of corroboration of self-reports
7. small sample size and poor follow-up response rate
8. poorly specified diagnostic, treatment, and outcome criteria

To begin with, an adequate discussion of the controversy is impossible without an understanding of the individual and environmental factors that motivates an individual to seek compensation. Two percent of the total industrial work force suffers a compensable back injury every year [50]. Compensation is merely one form of secondary gain, which is usually determined by several psychosocial variables including the patient's standard of living, age, physical and mental condition, responsibilities, job performance and relationship with his or her employer. Other kinds of gain might be psychological gratification, whereby disability encourages the love and attention of others, or physical gratification, where an aging employee experiencing increasing difficulty in performing his/her work tasks might use disability as a an excuse for reassignment to a less demanding duty. If return to the workplace requires a job change inconsistent with the ideas, goals, or customs of the patient and family, unspoken resistance may present as increased pain behavior, somatic focus, and unwillingness to explore work options.

Compensation is sometimes perceived by the employee as the most obvious means of retribution for previous injustices suffered at the hands of an indifferent, uncaring employer who rarely appreciated the employee's undervalued efforts. Work disatisfaction is another factor. Bigos et al. established a correlation between incidence of back injuries and poor employee appraisal rating performed by the employee's supervisor within six months before the injury [51]. Furthermore, Magora believes that work disatisfaction increases the likelihood of a worker filing a compensation claim [52]. Those who were previously performing unfulfilling or menial jobs, or experiencing stress or discontent in the workplace, may prefer to continue collecting an often substantial portion of their previous salary rather than return to work. This desire could be compounded by a low educational level or language difficulties which limit alternative vocational opportunity.

Adversarial relations during the disability period only add to the sense of righteous indignation the employee feels, intensifying the desire to correct the perceived wrongs by prolonging his symptoms for secondary gain. In addition to the genuine distress the individual must feel when forced to prove he is actually injured, the process of litigation may reinforce and aggravate the patient's pain behavior, and thus provide additional incentive to maximize the final settlement. Consequently, the pain behavior develops into a learned response and becomes the disability for which the patient is seeking compensation. Often, the outcome of compensation can not be mediated in-house, but rather in the courtroom: "Such prolonged legal sparring, which often involves an attack on the patient's validity, may serve to create a more firmly fixed symptom complex than would occur in a nonadversary situation"[3]. The entire process is generally characterized by suspicion, resentment, and frustration for all concerned. Some doctors simply reinforce these emotions with their belief that compensation patients are untreatable, more likely to exhibit abnormal personality traits, and inherently prone to exaggerate pain severity and disability to maximize the damages awarded.

There is some factual basis for this critical stereotype. It can be argued, for instance, that improved worker's compensation benefits result in additional claim filings and injuries. A clear example of this trend was observed by Robertson et al. in an evaluation of the effects of workers' compensation on work injuries from 1973 to 1980 [53]. When exposure to hazard and worker attributes were controlled, the authors found that changes in injury rates were primarily explained by increases in workers' compensation benefits. The surge in reported injuries corresponded quite well with the trend during the seventies toward increasing disability payments at a rate substantially greater than inflation. In those states where payments were twice the inflation rate, lost work days from injury claims increased by 600 to 900 days for each industrial grouping. If this report is an accurate representation of national trends, it should come as no surprise that from 1971 to 1981 the population disabled by low back pain increased at a rate 14 times that of the growth of the U.S. population itself, a rate of increase far greater than that of any other disease in America [54].

A linear relationship between the level of benefits and the duration of back-related work loss was noted by Worral, based upon three studies using data from the National Council on Compensation Insurance [55-57]. The data indicated that an increase of 10% in compensation benefits translated to a two to five day increase in time off work. According to Walsh, "the greater the financial compensation, the longer individuals remain off work... Economic incentives are inherent in the workers' compensation program, and it appears that the average worker responds to such incentives" [58].

However, other dissenting reports do not justify the stereotype of compensation-driven chronic pain patient, as the reader will recognize in the studies to follow. A comparison between compensation patients and non-compensation patients was undertaken by Leavitt et al. to evaluate the distribution of psychologic disturbance, organic status and pain report characteristics [59]. The group consisted of 85 patients receiving compensation and 176 patients not on compensation and with no pending claims. The authors found that the compensation group experienced 12% more cases of unconfirmed organic disease, but the difference was not judged statistically significant. With respect to psychologic disturbance, 30% of the patients in each group tested positive on the Low Back Classification Scale, casting doubt on the belief that psychologic disturbance either predisposes patients to seek compensation or is exacerbated by compensation. The most important difference was seen in the description of pain characteristics, where compensation patients with clear organic findings used 43% more words to describe their pain and endorsed more pain qualities on five independent dimensions of pain measuring sensory discomfort. Because the two groups not demonstrating organic etiology described pain in essentially the same terms, the authors put forth the following hypothesis: "Compensation seems to exacerbate several components of pain only among patients with clear signs of organic disease who are also not psychologically disturbed. That is, the effects of compensation are apparent only among those patients about whom there is least reason to suspect malingering... Little justification was found for the atmosphere of suspicion that surrounds patients on compensation who have no evidence of organic disease." It is speculated that these compensation patients describe more pain because they might believe that the injury is not regarded seriously by the employer, thus they feel the need to insist upon the existence of signs and symptoms of an actual injury.

A similar study along the same lines was conducted by Mendelson to evaluate the pain reports and illness behavior among 89 litigants (71 of which complained of chronic low back pain) and 37 patients with chronic low back pain not related to a compensable injury [60]. Results were based upon several psychological test, including the Eysenck Personality Inventory, the Zung Self-Rating Depression Scale, and the State-Trait Anxiety Inventory. Particular emphasis was placed on the Illness Behavior Questionnaire, a profile of attitudes toward illness, and communication of affect, denial and irritability. No differences between the two groups were noted on any of the measures of pain severity, although the compensation patients did have a significant elevation of mean score on the depression scale of the psychological tests. The groups differed very little with regard to illness behavior, in term of hypochondriasis, disease convicton, somatic or psychological attitude to symptoms, and affective inhibition. Mendelson concludes: "The assumption — I hate to use the term prejudice -- that litigants exaggerate their symptoms has not been confirmed by the use of scales which provided a quantifiable measure of pain and illness behavior."

Melzack utilized a different measuring stick to evaluate the psychological differences between 81 compensation and non-compensation patients suffering from chronic low back pain [61]. The results of the McGill Pain Questionnaire (a list of adjectives describing pain severity) and MMPI indicated some unusual findings. There was a remarkable consistency with which patients described their pain, regardless of whether or not they were receiving financial compensation. With one exception, every word chosen by 30% or more of the compensation patients was also chosen by 30% or more of the non-compensation patients. Among the more notable differences, 41% of the non-compensation patients considered their pain as "sickening," versus only 15% of the compensation group. Additionally, compensation patients saw on average fewer doctors and rated the overall intensity of pain as significantly lower than the non-compensation group. Melzack proposes that the difference in scores could be the result of greater financial worries for the non-compensation patients, reflected in their higher affective and evaluative scores. Both groups demonstrated high scores on the MMPI "neurotic triad" (depression, hysteria, and hypochondriasis) when compared to the normal population, but showed no differences between compensation and non-compensation patients. In response to the proponents of the "compensation neuroses" theory, Melzack concludes: "Compensation is not a cause of pain, though it is often referred to that way... To select a single factor as the sole cause represents a failure to recognize the complexity of pain. This does not mean that malingerers or neurotics do not exist. It suggests instead that they may be relatively rare and that unfortunate patients have been misdiagnosed, mistreated and allowed to suffer under the shroud of unfair labels instead of receiving appropriate therapy."

The previous three studies suggest that patients receiving compensation are no more emotionally disturbed by back pain severity and chronic disability than are patients not receiving compensation, although both groups are more distressed than the general public. Some recent reports dispute this finding. For instance, Sternbach asserted that the MMPI scores of compensation patients showed elevated scores on hypochondriasis, depression, and hysteria scales when compared to patients not receiving compensation [27]. The elevated "neurotic triad" scores were considered remarkably similar to patients with non-organic low back pain, lending persuasive support to the intuitive linkage between compensation and non-organic status. The author described this trend as a "clear potentiation of the psychosphysiological symptoms by the litigation factor." Bochner noted that patients with back pain involved in litigation show emotional symptoms which he attributed to "the fight for compensation," and emphasized the importance of these symptoms in the overall management of the patient [62].

Another debate about the compensation patient as a malingerer or legitimate pain sufferer is not over the psychological status of such individuals, but rather their response to treatment [63]. According to Mendelson, there is a "general impression that patients involved in litigation do not improve until the compensation claim has been finalized, and this has been at times used as a criterion when evaluating patient suitability for treatment." In other words, certain hospitals, back schools, or pain clinics will not admit a patient receiving compensation because the probability of treatment failure is too high. A 1983 review concluded that the results of the studies published up to that time were in general agreement that patients receiving compensation and/or involved in litigation had a worse prognosis than those non-compensation patients with similar complaints [64].

Consistent with this viewpoint is a study by Sander et al. of the influence of compensation on recovery from work-related back pain in the railroad industry [65]. Workers receiving compensation showed dramatically slower recovery than those not receiving compensation. The average work loss after back injury was 14.9 months for the 35 patients injured on the job (thus eligible for compensation) compared to 3.6 months for patients injured away from the workplace. Even when employees were matched for age, type of injury, and severity of injury, those injured while on duty were off work for an average of 14.2 months, versus 4.9 months for the employees injured off duty. Moreover, the average time off work in patients undergoing surgical repair of herniated discs was 9.3 months for on-duty injuries and 4.4 months for off-duty injuries.

Verification of these results are reported by Hudgins in a study where 73 patients receiving compensation and 73 non-compensation patients were carefully matched for physical signs, type of disc abnormality found at surgery, myelographic findings, duration of symptoms, sex, age, and estimated degree of physical stress at work [66]. The patients receiving compensation reported one-third as many excellent results (no residual symptoms and working without impairment) and four times as many poor results. While 100% of the non-compensation patients were working one year post-operatively, 77% of the compensation patients were employed. Additionally, surgical failure (no pain relief) was three times as prevalent among the compensation patients.

Treatment failure associated with compensation and litigation is not limited to surgical outcome, but includes many different types of rehabilitative modalities. A study of 509 patients by Krusen et al. found that of the 272 compensation claimants, 56% were rated as improved when discharged from physical therapy, compared with 89% of improved patients in a group of 237 not receiving compensation [67]. The poor outcome among the compensation patients comes despite the fact that they received twice as many therapy treatments as the non-compensation patients. Similar results were observed by Warfield et al. during epidural steriod injection of 161 patients with lumbar radiculopathy, finding 52% of the compensation patients reporting improvement after injection, versus 68% of the non-compensation patients [68]. Concerning the comparative efficacy of nerve blocks, Hammonds found that 69% of the non-compensation patients made significant increases in their functional performance, while only 43% of the compensation patients showed similar improvement [69]. In another study, Trief et al. reported that patients without pending litigation obtained significantly greater benefits from a six-week behavioral treatment program, based upon changes in MMPI scales and two of three behavioral measures of physical mobility [70].

A careful consideration of the preceding reports has lead Walsh et al. to the following conclusion: "Most current evidence suggests that the system of disability compensation in the United States does increase the frequency of certain types of disability claims and contribute to delayed recovery from low back pain. Recovery following conservative therapy, back surgery, and chronic pain rehabilitation programs all appear to be influenced by concurrent disability claims or compensation... It does appear that compensation factors may delay recovery, prolong symptoms, and reinforce sick role behavior" [58].

Although there are many studies available that demonstrate conclusively that the compensation patient responds less favorably than other patients to a wide variety of treatments (especially surgery), a few reports have indicated that compensation has little or no impact upon successful rehabilitation. With the recent focus in back treatment on early intervention, rehabilitation and rapid return of the employee to the workplace, reports of poor treatment outcome with compensation patients are becoming less apparent. For instance, no statistical difference was found by Raaf when compensation patients were compared to non-compensation patients following operation for herniated lumbar disc [71]. White randomly assigned 194 patients receiving compensation for low back injuries to either treatment by the family doctor or at a rehabilitation center, hypothesizing that if compensation had an adverse effect on treatment outcome, then there would be little difference between the two groups [72]. Instead, the back clinic proved to be two and one-half more effective than the family doctor (improvement in 42% versus 16%). The author concluded that compensation payment for disability did not delay recovery to a significant degree. A study by Ganora of 150 compensable back cases referred to a rehabilitation center documented a return-to-work rate of 61% [73]. This was a considerable achievement, given that 66% of the patients were not working prior to admission. Post-treatment results demonstrated that 75% of the patients with pain duration shorter than three months were back on the job, as were 50% of those with pain in excess of three months. Early rehabilitation was emphasized as a primary reason for the dramatic success of the program, claiming that "the pessimism generally expressed in the management of work-related back injury is unfounded."

Aronoff et al. has identified the compensation patient most likely to respond favorably to treatment, based upon the various physical, psychological, and environmental factors implicated in chronic back pain [1]. These authors feel probability of successful rehabilitation of the compensation patient is greatest under the following circumstances:

1. early intervention and rehabilitation,
2. positive hospital course: high motivation, effective mastery of pain, and success in stress reduction strategies,

3. positive work history in which employment offered purpose and satisfaction; high incentive to return to work,
4. no major psychopathology
5. no narcotic/analgesic dependency,
6. primary/secondary/tertiary gain factors not operative in perpetuating pain syndrome,
7. no litigation, and
8. expeditious return to work/school after hospital discharge.

The incorporation of return-to-work as a major objective of treatment was evaluated by Catchlove et al. and found to be an integral component of effective therapy [74]. Patients were assigned to one of two treatment groups: twenty patients were treated without any specific instruction concerning resumption of work, while 27 were administered similar treatment which also included a specific return to work emphasis. Patients in the group directed to return to work were informed upon admission that they would need to resume work within one to two months, and this was part of the initial treatment "contract." The staff continually reinforced the concept by actively initiating return to work discussions and by guiding patients in setting work goals according to their disabilities. At post-treatment, 59% of the "instruction" group returned to their jobs, whereas only 25% of the group not receiving instruction had resumed work. Long-term follow-up also indicated that working patients showed a sense of satisfaction and increased independence.

Employment status among compensable (and litigant) chronic pain patients was also analyzed by Dworkin et al., who hypothesized that poor treatment outcome was strongly related to the fact that such patients are less likely to be working than patients not receiving compensation and without pending litigation [75]. The study examined the relationships among compensation, litigation, employment, and short- and long-term therapy results among 454 chronic pain patients. The nature of chronic illness among the participants was not limited to back patients but included a wide variety of painful syndromes: cancer, neck and shoulder pain, various myofascial syndromes, among other pathologies. Treatment utilized a multimodal approach, individualized for each patient based on history, physical examination, and diagnostic results. Demographic analysis indicated that compensation patients were significantly more likely to be male, younger in age, and not be working at the time of their evaluation than were non-compensation patients. Patients in receipt of compensation had a poorer short-term treatment response than their non-compensated counterparts, while patients working at the time of their initial evaluation had a better response to treatment than unemployed workers.

A stepwise multiple regression analysis predicting short-term treatment outcome revealed that employment was the only statistically significant predictor of outcome. Neither compensation or pending litigation was shown associated with poorer outcome. As for long-term treatment response, only employment at the time of initial evaluation significantly predicted outcome. The authors believe that employment status could explain the tremendous variability of reported treatment outcome among patients in receipt of compensation or with pending legislation, as the percentage of compensation patients that also work varies tremendously between published reports. Based upon the results of this study, the authors strongly recommend that treatment programs should further emphasize patient education, counseling, vocational intervention, or other forms of instruction designed to return the worker to employment.

Rather than employment as the key determinant of treatment outcome, the most pessimistic physicians and lawyers argue that if compensation delays return to gainful employment, then most claimants might return to work shortly after finalization of the compensation claim. It is suggested that finalization of the compensation claim is the most effective remedy of "compensation neuroses," leading to complete physical recovery. Evidence supporting this viewpoint is extremely scarce. The only example we could find in the literature was a report of a follow-up of 17 patients diagnosed with "compensation hysteria" which found that of the seven patients successfully traced following settelment, six recovered within a short period of time and returned to work. The seventh patient continued to receive a pension for several years until it was withdrawn, prompting his resumption of work as well. This kind of experience appears to be the exception to the rule, if current research on the topic is any indication.

References

1. Aronoff GM, McAlary PW, Witkower A, Berdell MS: Pain treatment programs: Do they return workers to the workplace? Occup Med: State of the Art Reviews 3(1):123-135, 1988.
2. Waddell G, Main CJ, Morris EW, Di Paola M, Gray ICM: Chronic low back pain, psychologic distress, and illness behavior. Spine 9(2):209-213, 1984.
3. Finnesson BE: Low back pain. J.B. Lippincott, Philadelphia, 1980.
4. Sternbach RA: Psychological factors in pain. Adv Res Therapy 1:293, 1976.
5. Peterson LE: A cognitive-behavioral perspective in the assessment and treatment of chronic low back pain. In Chronic Low Back Pain. Stanton-Hicks M, Boas R (eds.). Raven Press, New York, 1982.
6. Finnesson B: The Psychology of Low Back Dysfunction, from Low Back Pain. J.B. Lippincott, Philadelphia, PA, 1980.
7. Watkins RG, Collis JS, Jr.: Lumbar discectomy and laminectomy - Principles and techniques in spine surgery. Aspen, 1987.

8. Pilowsky I, Spence ND: Illness behavior syndromes associated with intractable pain. Pain 2:61-71, 1976.
9. Engle G: Psychogenic pain and the pain-prone patient. Am J Med 26:89-918, 1959.
10. Clawson DK: Psychologic aspects of pain. From Ruge D, Wiltse LL: Spinal Disorders - Diagnosis and Treatment. Lea & Febiger, Philadelphia, 1977.
11. Leavitt F, Garron DC: Patterns of psychological disturbance and pain report in patients with low back pain. J of Psychosomatic Res 26(3):301-307, 1982.
12. Garron DC, Leavitt F: Chronic low back pain and depression. J of Clin Psych 39(4):487-493, 1983.
13. Sternbach RA, Wolf SR, Murphy RW, Akeson WH: Aspects of chronic low back pain. Psychosom 14:52-56, 1973.
14. Ward NG, Bloom VL, Freidel RO: The effectiveness of tricyclic antidepressants in the treatment of co-existing pain and depression. Pain 7:331-341, 1979.
15. Sternbach RA, Timmermans G: Personality changes associated with reduction of pain. Pain 1:177-181, 1975.
16. Merskey H: The characteristics of persistent pain in psychological illness. J Psychosom Res 9:291-298, 1965.
17. Beals RK, Hickman NW: Industrial injuries of the back and extremities. J of Bone Joint Surg 54A:1593-1611, 1972.
18. Freedman DX, Smith RJ, Lehmann, et al: Depression today. Part I. Recognizing and diagnosing depression. 31st Winter Scientific Meeting of AMA, December, 1977, New York, CME Communications, Inc., 1978.
19. Vallfors B: Acute, subacute and chronic low back pain, clinical symptoms, absenteeism and working environment . Scan J Rehabil Med 11:1-98, 1985.
20. Hanvik LJ: MMPI profiles used in patients with low back pain. J Consult Psychol 15:350-353, 1951.
21. Freeman C, Calsyn D, Louks J: The use of MMPI with low back pain patients. J Clin Psychol 32:294-298, 1976.
22. Merskey H, Boyd D: Emotional adjustment and chronic pain. Pain 5:173-178, 1978.
23. Carr JE, Brownsberger CN, Rutherford RC: Characteristics of symptom-matched psychogenic and real pain patients of the MMPI. Proc. 74th Ann Conv Amer Psycho Assoc. 1966:215- 216.
24. Lair CV, Trapp EP: The differential diagnostic value of MMPI with somatically disturbed patients. J Clin Psychol 18:146-147, 1962.
25. McCreary C, Turner J, Dawson E: Differences between functional versus organic low back pain patients. Pain 4:73-78, 1977.

26. Woodforde J, Merskey H: Personality traits of patients with chronic pain. J Psychosom Res 16:167-172, 1972.
27. Sternbach RA, Wolf SR, Murphy RW, Adeson WH: Traits of pain patients: The low back "loser". Psychosomatics 14:226-229, 1973.
28. Waddell G, Main CJ: Chronic backache, distress, illness behavior and surgery. Acta Orthop Belgica 53(2):265-266, 1987.
29. Calliet R: Low back pain syndrome. FA Davis, Philadelphia, 1981.
30. Linton SJ: A critical review of behavioral treatments for chronic benign pain other than headache. Br J of Clin Psych 21:321-337, 1982.
31. Fordyce WE, Brockway JA, Bergman JA, Spengler D: Acute back pain: A control-group comparison of behavioral vs traditional management methods. J of Behav Med 9(2):127-140, 1986.
32. Anderson TP, Cole TM, Gullickson G, Hudgens A, Roberts AH: Behavior modification of chronic pain: a treatment program by a multidisciplinary team. Clin Orthop 129:96-100, 1977.
33. Cairns D, Thomas L, Mooney V, Pace JB: A comprehensive treatment approach to chronic low back pain. Pain 2:301-308, 1976.
34. Turk DC, Flor H: Etiological theories and treatments for chronic back pain. II. Psychological models and interventions. Pain 19:209-233, 1984.
35. Janus L: Psychophysiologische Untersuchungen bei funkteionellen Muskelverspannungen im Nackenbereich. In: Weintraub A, Battegay R, Beck D, Kaganas G, Labhardt F, Muller W. (Eds). Psychosomatische Schmerzsyndrome des Bewegungsapparates Schwabe. Basel, 1975, pp. 47-91.
36. Holmes TH, Wolff HG: Life situations, emotions, and bachache. Proc As Res Nerv Ment Dis 29:750-772, 1950.
37. Dorpat TL, Holmes TH: Backache and muscle tension origin. In: WS Kroger (ed)., Psychosomatic Obstetrics, Gynecology and Endocrinology. Thomas, Springfield, IL. 1962.
38. Nouwen A: EMG biofeedback used to reduce standing levels of paraspinal muscle tension in chronic low back pain. Pain 17:353-360, 1983.
39. Nouwen A: Comparison of EMG biofeedback and electrotherapy in chronic low back pain. bibliography needed.
40. Jones AL, Wolf SL: Treating chronic low back pain -- EMG biofeedback training during movement. Phys Ther 60:58-63, 1980.
41. Flor H, Haag G, Turk DC, Koehler H: Efficacy of EMG biofeedback, pseudotherapy, and conventional medical treatment for chronic rheumatic back pain. Pain 17:21-31, 1983.
42. Peterson LE: A cognitive-behavioral perspective in the assessment and treatment of chronic low back pain. From Stanton-Hicks M, Boas R (Eds.): Chronic Low Back Pain. Raven Press, New York, 1982, pp.133-143.

43. Cohen MJ, Heinrich RL, Collins GA, Bonebakker AD: Group outpatient physical or behavioral therapy for chronic low back pain. Paper presented at the Annual Meeting of the American Pain Society, New York, September 1980.
44. Turner JA: Comparison of group progressive-relaxation training and cognitive-behavioral group therapy for chronic low back pain. J Consult Clin Psychol 50(5):757-765, 1982.
45. Aronoff GM: The role of the pain center in the treatment of intractable suffering and disability resulting from chronic pain. Seminol Neurol 3(4):377, 1983.
46. Gottlieb H, Strite LC, Koller R, Madorsky A, Hockersmith V, Kleeman M, Wagner J: Comprehensive rehabilitation of patients having chronic low back pain. Arch Phys Med Rehab 58:101-108, 1977.
47. Kennedy F: The mind of the injured worker: its effect on disability periods. Compens Med 1:19-24, 1946.
48. Rothman RH, Simeone FA: The Spine. Philadelphia, WB Saunders, 1982.
49. Snook SH, et al: A study of three preventative approaches to low back injury. J Occup Med 20:478-481, 1978.
50. Bond MB: Low back injuries in industry. Indust Med Surg 39:204-208, 1970.
51. Bigos SJ, Spengler DM, Martin NA, et al: Back injury in industry: a retrospective study. III. Employee related factors. Spine 11:252-256, 1986.
52. Magora A: Investigation of the relation between low back pain and occupation. V. Psychological Aspects. Scand J Rehab Med 5:191, 1973.
53. Robertson LS, Keeve JP: Worker injuries: The effect of workers' compensation and OSHA inspections. Health Politics, Policy and Law 8:581-597, 1983.
54. National Center for Health Statistics: Series 10, No. 134. Prevalence of selected impairment, US - 1977. DHHS. Publication (PHS), Hyattsville, MD, 1985.
55. Worral JD, Appel D: The wage replacement rate and benefit utilization in workers' compensation insurance. J Risk Insur 49-361-371, 1982.
56. Worral JD, Appel D: The impact of workers' compensation benefits on low back claims. In Hadler NM (ed): Clinical Concepts in Regional Musculoskeletal Illness. Orlando, Grune and Stratton, 1987.
57. Worral JD, Butler RJ: Benefits and claim duration. In Worall JD, Appel D (eds): Workers' Compensation Benefits: Adequacy, Equity and Efficiency. Ithaca, ILR Press, 1985, pp. 57-70.
58. Walsh NE, Dumitru D: The influence of compensation on recovery from low back pain. Occup Med: State of the Art Reviews 3(1):109-121, 1988.
59. Leavitt F, Garron DC, McNeill TW, Whisler WW: Organic status, psychological disturbance, and pain report characterstics in low back pain patients on compensation. Spine 7(4):398-402, 1982.

60. Mendelson G: Illness behaviour, pain and personal injury litigation. Psych Med 5(1):39-49, 1987.
61. Melzack R, Katz J, Jeans ME: The role of compensation in chronic pain: Analysis using a new method of scoring the McGill pain questionnaire. Pain 23:101-112, 1985.
62. Bochner AK: Psychiatric aspects of back injuries. In Schroeder O (ed): The Back: a Law-Medicine Problem. Cincinnati, Anderson, 1965.
63. Mendelson G: Chronic pain and compensation: A review. J of Pain and Symp Manag 1(3):135-144, 1986.
64. Mendelson G: The effect of compensation and litigation on disability following compensable injuries. American J of Forensic Psych 4:97-112, 1983.
65. Sander RA, Meyers JE: The relationship of disability to compensation status in railroad workers. Spine 11:141-143, 1984.
66. Hudgins WR: Compensation and success of lumbar disc surgery. Texas Med 70:62-65, 1974.
67. Krusen EM, Ford DE: Compensation factor in low back injuries. JAMA 166:1128-1133, 1958.
68. Warfield CA, Crews DA: Work status and response to epidural steroid injection. J Occup Med 29:315-316, 1987.
69. Hammonds W, Brena SF, Unikel IP: Compensation for work related injuries in rehabilitation of patients with chronic pain. Southern Med J 71:664-666, 1978.
70. Trief P, Stein N: Pending litigation and rehabilitation outcome of chronic back pain. Arch Phys Med Rehabil 66:95-99, 1985.
71. Raaf J: Some observations regarding 905 patients operated upon for protruded lumbar intervertebral disc. Amer J Surg 97:388-397, 1959.
72. White AWM: Low back pain in men receiving workmen's compensation. Canad Med Ass J 95:50-56, 1966.
73. Ganora A: Comprehensive back pain rehabilitation in 150 compensable low back injuries: methods and initial results. Abstracts of the Annual Science Meeting of the Australian Pain Society. Sydney, Feb. 1984(24).
74. Catchlove R, Cohen K: Directive approach with workmen's compensation patients. Advances in Pain Research and Therapy 5:913-918, 1985.
75. Dworkin RH, Handlin DS, Richlin DM, Brand L, Vannucci C: Unraveling the effects of compensation, litigation, and employment on treatment response in chronic pain. Pain 23:49-59, 1985.

Glossary

Anaphylactic - Immediate severe allergic reaction.
Annulus - Outer part of the intervertebral disc.
Anteroposterior - Pertaining to the front and rear.
Anthropometric - Measurement of proportions of the human body.
Arachnoiditis - Inflammatory disease leading to scarring which binds the nerve roots.
Arthropathy - Any disease affecting a joint.
Articular - Pertaining to a joint.

Biofeedback - The process of providing an individual with visual or auditory evidence of the status of an unconscious body function.

Chemonucleolysis - Treatment of intervertebral disc lesions by the intradiscal injection of an agent, most commonly chymopapain.
Claudication - Cramping leg pain
Chymopapain - A papaya enzyme that dissolves intervertebral disc nucleus.
Compensation neurosis - The tendency of individuals to maintain various symptoms which originally occured as the result of injury, as a defense against losing the various secondary gains obtained from the injury, particularly monetary.
Conversion 'V' - A specific pattern on the MMPI test profile which is believed to be correlated with an emotional component in an individual expressing physical pain. The patient emphasizes, but fails to show real concern about somatic symptoms. Depression or anxiety is conspicuously absent.

Disc degeneration - Loss of structural and functional integrity of the disc.
Discectomy - Excision of all or part of the intervertebral disc.
Discitis - Inflammatory disease of the disc.
Discogenic - Pain caused by derangement of an intervertebral disc.
Discography - The introduction of radio-opaque fluid into the nucleus pulposus for purposes of identifying disc configuration.
Dorsal - Related to back, posterior.

Electromyograph (EMG) - Recording of electrical output of the contraction of a muscle.
Endplate - The part of a vertebra where it joins the intervertebral disc.
Epidemiology - The study of disease (epidemics) among populations.
Ergonomics - Science that seeks to adapt working conditions to suit the worker.
Etiology - Study of the causes of disease.

Facets - A pair of joints, at each vertebral level, essential for spine stabilization and bending capacity.
Facet arthritis - Degenerative changes of the facet joints characterized by cartilage thinning and osteophyte formation.
Facet tropism - Asymmetrical orientation of the right and left facet joints.
Fibrosus - Formation of fibrous tissue.
Fusion - Surgically connecting two or more bones together to form one unit.

Herniated disc - Displacement of nucleus pulposus and other disc components beyond the normal confines of the annulus.
A. Protrusion - Displaced material casuses a bulge in the annulus, but no material escapes through the annular fibers.
B. Extrusion - Displaced material presents in the spinal canal through disrupted annular fibers, but remains connected to material persisting within the disc.
C. Sequestration - Nuclear material escapes into the spinal canal as a free fragment(s) which may migrate to other locations.

Idiopathic - Denoting a primary disease of unknown origin.
Ischemic - Relating to lack of blood supply.

Laminectomy - Removal of a lamina from its superior to its inferior margin.
Lordosis - Curvature of spinal column as seen from the side (S-curve).
Lumbar - Pertaining to last five vertebra of the spine.

Nucleus pulposus - The central, viscous portion of the intervertebral disc.
Neuroses - An emotional illness without marked losss of contact with reality.

Orthosis - Orthopedic device for supporting the spine (e.g. brace or corset).
Osteoarthritis - Degenerative arthritis affecting many joints.
Osteopenia - Any state in which bone mass is reduced below normal.
Osteoporosis - Diminution in both the mineral and matrix components of bone.

Psuedoarthrosis - A defect in bone secondary to failure of union in either a bone or bone graft.
Psychophysiologic disorder - Physical symptoms that are caused by emotioal factors.

Radiopaque - Impenetrable by x-rays
Radiculitis - Inflammation of a spinal nerve in the spinal canal or neural canal.
Radiculopathy - Non-inflammatory abnormality of a spinal nerve in the spinal canal or neural foramen resulting in neurological deficit.

Sacroiliac - Relating to the joint between the pelvis and vertebral column.
Sagittal - Anatomic plane passing vertically through the body from front to back.

Scoliosis - Abnormal curvature of vertebral column.
Secondary gain - An external situational gain derived from any illness.
Segmental instability - An abnormal, excessive motion between two adjacent vertebrae, associated with painful symptoms.
Spasm - Involuntary muscle contraction.
Spinal stenosis - Reduction in the size of the spinal canal.
Spondylitis - An inflammatory disease of the spine.
Spondylolisthesis - Anterior displacement of a vertebra on the adjacent vertebra.
Spondylolysis - A defect in the vertebra (pars interarticularis).
Spondylosis - Degenerative disease of both the disc and the facet joints.
Subluxation - Partial dislocation of a joint.

Traction spur - A bony protrusion appearing on the anterolateral surface of the vertebral body near the body margin which arises as a result of disc degeneration.

Index